T0297026

Hate and Love in
Psychoanalytical Institutions

Hate and Love in Psychoanalytical Institutions

The Dilemma of a Profession

Jurgen Reeder

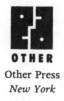

OTHER
Other Press
New York

Library of Congress Cataloging-in-Publication Data

Reeder, Jurgen, 1947–
    Hate and love in psychoanalytical institutions : the dilemma of a profession / by Jurgen Reeder.
        p. cm.
Includes bibliographical references (p.   ) and index.
        ISBN 1-59051-065-8 (pbk.)
        1. Psychoanalysis—Practice.   2. Psychoanalysis—Training of.
3. Psychoanalysis—Study and teaching.   4. Superego.   5. Love-hate relationships.   I. Title.
        RC506 .R3864 2004
        616.89'17–dc22

                                                                    2003024323

Contents

Preface   ix

1. Introduction   1

   Perspectives   5
   Presentation   7
   The Significance of This Study   9
   A Short Itinerary   10

2. Psychoanalysis as Praxis: A Personal View   13

   Dialogical Interpreting   17
      Communication, Transference, and
         Countertransference   18
      The Matrix of Transference   21
      Vignette   23
      With Evenly Suspended Attention   27
      The Process of Clinical Reflection   30
      Hope and Faith   32
      The Faithfulness of Truth   34
   On Theoretical Work   35
      Three Levels of Psychoanalytic Knowing   37
      Construction: Clinical Theory   38
      Assimilation   42
      Construction: Metapsychology   45
      The Experiential Basis of Theoretical Work   48
      Inventing the Analysand Anew   50

3. The Epochs of the Psychoanalytic Institution   53

   The Berlin Institute   56
      The Training System   59
      International Developments   64
   The Three Epochs of the Psychoanalytic Institution   66
   Psychoanalysis and Psychiatry   72
      The Demise of the APA as a Medical Bastion   77

4. Central Functions in Psychoanalytic Training   81

   The Selection of Candidates   85
   Didactic Analysis, Training Analysis,
      Personal Analysis   94
      The Therapeutic Aim   95
      Selection and Evaluation   101
      The Transmission of an Experience   106
      The Normalization of the Analyst   112
   The Supervised Cases   118
      The Pedagogic Conflict   121
      The Syncretism of Supervision   125
      Intimacy and Control   128
      The Supervisor's Function as Mentor   135
   The Theoretical Seminars   140

5. The Superego Complex   145

   Concepts and Their Use   153
   A State within the State   154
      An Institution, Not an Organization   155
      Incestuous Ties, Oedipal Relations,
         and Power   160
   The Superego Complex   165
      The Immanent Pedagogy of the
         Psychoanalytic Institution   166
      Superego and Ego Ideal   168
      Fueled by Hate   170
      The Superego Complex as the Culture of Hate   173

Externalized Hate 176
Paranoia, Hostility, and the Pursuit
of the Psychopath 178
Effects on Theoretical Work 188
The Psychoanalyst's Inner Career 197
Prescription and Ethos 197
Decisive Years 201
Orthos Doxa 206
The Tyranny of Interpretations 208
The Hermeneutics of Suspicion 210
From Superego to Ego Ideal 213

6. Concluding Reflections 221

What Is to Be Done? 224
Abolish the Training Analyst Institution 228
In Defense of a Wholly Independent
Personal Analysis 230
Strengthen the Supervisory Function 233
Make Room for Theoretical Work and
Necessary Research 235
Make Training More Accessible 239
Make Power More Transparent 240
Psychoanalysis and Its Uncertain Future 241

End Notes 249

References 277

Index 301

About the Author 309

Abstract 310

Preface

Friends and helpful colleagues are indispensable for anyone engaged in research and writing. During the period that this project developed, a number of people have afforded their reactions, suggestions, analyses, criticism, and—not in the least—moral support. Had any of this been lacking, the book would surely be a weak shadow of what it has turned out to be. Therefore, gratitude is due.

Above all, I wish to thank the analysand I here call "Eva," who has allowed me, in Chapter 2, to include a reconstruction of the dialogue taking place during one of our sessions.

Hate and Love in Psychoanalytical Institutions has been generated under the auspices of a Swedish research program entitled "Transitions: Psychoanalytic Investigations into the Nature of Change." In that context, I have Iréne Matthis, Andrzej Werbart, Sonja Levander, and Gunnar Karlsson to thank for their views and inspiration during recurrent seminars, which, through the years, have become evermore important.

I also wish to thank Ulla-Britt Parment, Christer Sjödin, and Arne Jemstedt, all of whom, during the last year of my work, have read the text in its entirety and given feedback of a kind that has been necessary for me to finish the project.

My special appreciation goes to Charlotte Skawonius, who with unrelenting precision was always ready to convey how the text might be received by a nonpsychoanalytic audience. Likewise, I wish to thank John Swedenmark, who expressed very valuable views on Part 2 of Chapter 2.

Professors Birgitta Qvarsell and Arvid Löfberg at the Department of Education, Stockholm University, have provided both the program and my personal project with an abode at the university. The Swedish Council for Research in the Humanities and Social Sciences sponsored me to read, think, and write during the years 1995–1999. To all involved I wish to express my very deep gratitude for the confidence and generosity with which I have been received and supported.

I also wish to express my deeply felt gratitude to all those who have produced the evolving versions of *The PEP Archive* on CD-ROM, including more than 30,000 psychoanalytic articles from the six most prominent analytic publications in English, from their inception until 1998. Without access to the encyclopedic range of knowledge engraved on this little compact disk I would have produced a meager tome indeed.

During the course of my writing this book, preparatory work and "work in progress" have been published as articles in the Swedish journal *Divan* (Reeder 1998b, 1999), the first of which also appeared in English translation in the *International Forum of Psychoanalysis* (Reeder 1998c) and the second in the *International Journal of Psycho-Analysis* (Reeder 2002). In addition, two texts have been published in the internal *Bulletin of the Swedish Psychoanalytic Association* (Reeder 1998a,d). More or less modified, all these writings have been integrated into the final report. I should also mention that central aspects of Part 1 of Chapter 2 have previously appeared in Reeder 1996. I thank all the respective publishers for allowing me to include these texts in this book.

Finally, I wish to express my very sincere gratitude to Judy Cohen, who with the utmost care and sagacity has copyedited my translation during the first stages of production. Her assistance has definitely made my book a considerably more pleasant reading experience than it would have been otherwise.

Tomelilla, Sweden, March 1, 2004

I

INTRODUCTION

What follows is an investigation of a certain form of inhibiting structure that seems to arise easily within certain professional cultures. It seems to appear especially in cultures that are characterized by extensive specialization and hierarchization.

I have chosen to study this phenomenon by taking psychoanalysis as my example, primarily because analysis has been my professional habitat for almost thirty years. I began my training in 1973 and matriculated in 1979, when I was 32 years old. During the first eight years of independent work I was active in full-time private practice, exclusively with analytic patients whom I saw four times a week. This early period of my career consisted of what one at that time could expect the first years of a young psychoanalyst's professional life to contain: deep immersion in analytic work, many and extensive talks with colleagues, supervision individually and in different groups with visiting supervisors, trips to London for even more supervision, and—not least—studious reading. All of this aimed at getting a grip on what it is to be a psychoanalyst and developing the capacity to conduct a meaningful and convincing dialogue with my analysands.

In my previous book, *Reflecting Psychoanalysis* (Reeder 1996), I had described how after these initial years I was afflicted by a certain reticence in the clinical situation. I felt that what my chosen authorities and mentors wanted to convey was no longer adequate in my personal clinical experience. I no longer knew what to say to my analysands and often they would have to find their own answers as the intervals between my interventions grew longer.

At first I found no language for interpreting and understanding my predicament, but gradually I began thinking about it as the expression of two conflicts that were possibly interconnected. The first one could be formulated thusly: "With what legitimacy do I assume the right to interpret my fellow human being?" The second one had to do with an internalized system of ideals and norms and my endeavor to find my own way and my own voice as a practicing psychoanalyst. From this budding insight grew a hypothesis concerning what I initially called "the professional superego," a term chosen to designate both a prescriptive and an inhibiting instance, whose prescriptive aspect suggests what the analyst should know and be able to handle. In that respect, the professional superego supports the analyst's professional *ethos*. Its proscribing and inhibiting aspect, however, installs a vigilant eye that in turn will produce a more or less correct image of criticism or condemnation from the psychoanalytic community at large.[1]

The same year that I matriculated I was chosen to be a member of the board of the institute belonging to the Swedish Psychoanalytical Association (at that time called the Swedish Society for Holistic Psychotherapy and Psychoanalysis). To hold a position like that at such a young age is, as will be apparent from the account to follow, quite extraordinary. That it happened at all was because the society I belonged to was at that time only eleven years old, and of the group of people who had kept it going since it had been founded one had been forced to leave the society, one had died, and several had worn out their capacity as administrators. There were simply not enough experienced persons available to fill all the important posts. Still, the job had to be done, and I happened to be one of those who was assigned to do it.

I served the institute from 1979 to 1989, and during the greater part of that time I was its secretary. Apart from the purely secretarial aspects, which included the coordination of the institute's tasks, I was engaged in drawing up the institute's policy; partaking in the planning and administration of its five-year training; selecting candidates, supervisors, and training analysts; and evaluating candidates for the status of psychoanalyst. In addition, I worked on structuring the institute's organization and routines. In 1992 I was appointed to be a training analyst.

PERSPECTIVES

My research has always been related to my personal experience: I delve into that which does not leave me alone and demands an investigation. Therefore, the work of writing has always been the product of deep personal reflection. *Reflecting Psychoanalysis* was produced in an attempt to formulate a theoretical foundation for the kind of analytic work that gradually developed as my reticence abated and I found a style of conducting psychoanalysis that I could call my own. With this book I am investigating a complex that may have contributed to the kind of professional problem described above. In this, I benefit not only from more than twenty years of working as a psychoanalyst in private practice, but also from my time as an administrator within a psychoanalytic training institute.

When the idea of such an investigation began to develop and as I was formulating my application for a research grant (between 1994 and 1995), I regarded the superego issue almost wholly from an individual perspective. With such a view it was easy to slip into seeing the problem as a mere intrapsychic concern and something for the individual to come to grips with during the course of his career. One might think that my reticence problem would best be handled by my returning to the analytical couch. It is not improbable that something like that might have been beneficial, but then, it is rather uncertain whether a book like this would have been written.

The world of psychoanalysis is unique in how, with serious concern and ethical courage, it has conducted and published a wide-ranging internal discussion concerning the difficulties and problems inherent in the profession. This is so because the analytic project itself is to such a great extent an exercise in reflection, and with regard to their own practices, psychoanalysts simply continue to do what they do in their consulting rooms. As I started immersing myself in this vast literature I soon realized that it is quite insufficient to regard the professional superego as merely a private phenomenon. There also exists a corresponding institutional system within psychoanalytic organizations.

To encompass these two phenomena I will augment the concept of a "professional superego" with the "institutional superego system." Rather than being a characteristic of an individual psyche, the latter belongs to the culture of the profession itself. In the way that they interact, they form a whole, which I will call "the psychoanalytical superego complex." This complex has the same function as mentioned above, and thus is both prescriptive and inhibitory. But, because the superego in both of these aspects is effective through inculcating fear rather than inspiring love, the effect on the analyst will often be that his clinical and intellectual inventiveness is severely limited.

Psychoanalysis has helped people with serious personal problems to attain a better life. It has also been a source of deep satisfaction to its practitioners. However, analysts are dependent upon their institutions, and here lurks a danger that might affect the very activity itself. Through the presence of a superego complex the institutions have a tendency to betray the very analytical spirit for whose promotion they have been devised. One consequence of this is that they tend to fail when it comes to caring for their own. My main reason for pointing this out is not that I worry about the body of psychoanalysts. Rather it is psychoanalysis itself and its possibilities for growth and development that are my concern.

This is no isolated phenomenon among psychoanalysts. Precisely because of the way organizations and larger groups tend to structure themselves and function, tangibly destructive tendencies have a way of setting in and then being transmitted from one generation to another. This is not to deny the fact that individual organizations will, of course, differ in this respect, but all too often there lurks a threat to the integrity of the profession.

PRESENTATION

Following my original conceptions on the nature of the problem and my expectation that it would be difficult to find evidence of my hypothesis in the literature, I imagined that this book would be a rather small and handy volume. That is not how it turned out, however, and to my surprise and satisfaction my initial assumptions concerning an individual superego made it rather easy to discern what gradually developed into a more and more clear image of a greater complex. As my scope widened, so did the object of my research.

In what follows I aim to map, describe, and analyze the structure of the psychoanalytic superego complex: how it arises, how it works, how it is transmitted through the psychoanalytic training systems, and how it is maintained within analytic institutions. Against this background I will conclude by suggesting what might be done to minimize its destructive effects.

I will deal mainly with these phenomena as they have unfolded within the International Psychoanalytic Association (IPA), thus leaving out, for the most part, the corresponding developments within the International Federation of Psychoanalytic Societies (IFPS) and the Lacanian movement. To an even lesser extent do I touch upon conditions that might prevail within psychoanalytic groups existing outside of any superordinate organizations. There are three main reasons for this: (1) the IPA was founded in 1910, has existed longer than any other organization, and has the greatest number of members; (2) it has been necessary to limit my investigation and I deemed it natural to choose what is regarded as "mainstream" (which does not imply that I am thereby making any statement concerning what should be regarded as the "correct" way of conducting psychoanalysis); and (3) the issues and problems of interest here have been most extensively discussed and documented within the IPA. I will, however, make no attempt to delineate the history and conditions of any single psychoanalytic society, or of the origins and development within the two international organizations. Instead, I will limit my historical survey to discussing the evolution of the specifically psychoanalytic system of training that arose with the founding of an institute in Berlin during the twenties and that prevails largely unchanged in our time.[2]

The "empirical foundation" for my account consists mainly of the evidence given by those who have taken part in the internal discussions concerning difficulties and problems within the psychoanalytic movement. A considerable number of these contributions come from American psychoanalysts, a circumstance that might lead to the conclusion that what emerges here would not be applicable in other geographic areas, such as Europe or South America. My personal experience of working within a psychoanalytic institute in Sweden tells me, however, that the similarities are greater than the differences when it comes to the fundamental picture. Where I have stumbled upon decisive differences I have tried to compensate either with a comment or in the way a fact is presented.

The relative openness and critical courage of the Americans does not, however, imply that psychoanalysts there have necessarily been more successful in fighting and overcoming the very tendencies toward authoritarianism and organizational oppression that they criticize: the climate of debate is simply different. In a tragic way, all this openness, on both sides of the Atlantic, does not on the whole seem to have led to any greater changes. "Organizations are notorious for structuring themselves by rules, and the impact of this institutional structure on psychoanalysis and psychoanalytic education is well known. Change can occur, but institutionalization tends to oppose it" (Pulver 1985:175). This investigation aims at uncovering some central reasons things can turn out that way.

My report spans some eight decades and is more descriptive than analytical; my primary goal is not to explain phenomena but to depict them. In some sections a pronounced chronological way of approaching matters has been necessary, while simultaneously the temporal aspect may have been somewhat telescoped, with the effect that everything might seem to appear on one and the same temporal level. With this way of presenting things I want to demonstrate a general structure that is valid for a certain epoch and also how the institutional issues and problems of psychoanalysis have remained unchanged, to a surprising extent, during this phase of its evolution (which, I will maintain, began with the end of World War II and prevails to this day, although there are vital signs that changes are imminent).

In the central parts of my presentation—Chapters 3, 4, and 5— I rely to a great extent upon quotations (the "evidence" mentioned above), thereby giving space to the psychoanalytic movement's great variety of voices that have tried to analyze, criticize, support, or remedy the phenomena that I subsume under the label "the psychoanalytic superego complex."

I am aware that texts filled with excerpts from other authors' writings can make arduous reading when the reader is compelled to continually accommodate to new styles, idioms, and approaches. But because it has been my ambition to offer a broad picture of how things have been conceptualized and presented over the decades and to let as many witnesses as possible be heard, the avoidance of quotations would have counteracted one of the main objectives of the project. I have, however, made an effort to integrate the quotations with the text in a manner that I hope will facilitate reading.

THE SIGNIFICANCE OF THIS STUDY

To psychoanalysts and the even larger group of psychotherapists and counselors, a discussion of how the superego complex works would reasonably be of value for understanding and thinking about their professional identity and competence, as well as about the structure of training programs and postgraduate studies.

I also believe that the study of a phenomenon such as the super-ego complex can be of heuristic value to the exploration of other contexts in which a professional culture tends to collide with individual development. While active as a supervisor and discussion group leader within a welfare organization in Stockholm during the seventies, I observed similar phenomena among the social workers (it was most probably this experience that laid the foundation for my interest in conducting an investigation such as this one). Other professionals who might be inspired to undertake further research into their fields might be teachers, ministers, physicians, lawyers, academic researchers, and some leaders of corporations and larger institutions.

Of these areas not much will be said here. I can only hope that my own initiative and to some extent my heuristic model can be of help to others as they delve into their own professional lives. Of course, the methods employed must then be adapted to fit the reality to be investigated. One cannot, for example, expect to find the same unique collection of published analyses and critical comments that are connected with a superego complex that one can find in the psychoanalytic publications.

A SHORT ITINERARY

In Chapter 2, "Psychoanalysis as Praxis," I attempt to convey something of the realities of psychoanalytic work. I do this in the only way feasible to me: as a personal reflection upon some of its most significant aspects, a reasonably vivid picture of that very activity which it is the purpose of analytical institutions to safeguard and disseminate. This chapter not only provides a necessary background to the descriptions to follow, but also allows me to give vent to greater optimism than I feel I am able to do otherwise.

In Chapter 3, "The Epochs of the Psychoanalytic Institution," I describe the evolution of institutional structures, especially their development in Berlin during the twenties. In addition, I define the developmental phases of the psychoanalytic training system.

Chaper 4, "Central Functions in Psychoanalytic Training," describes the different elements of analytic training and their intended or unintended functions. Here the selection of candidates, the training analyses, the supervised cases, and the theoretical seminars are discussed.

Chapter 5, "The Superego Complex," describes, on the basis of what has been presented in Chapter 4, the superego complex as a general structure and how it manifests itself, both the form a superego system connected with the training analyst institution within psychoanalytical organizations takes, and as the analyst's professional superego.

In Chapter 6, "Concluding Reflections," I return to my personal reflections. Here I discuss some possible avenues for solving the problems connected with the analytic superego complex as well as the future of psychoanalysis within and outside the institutions.

With these chapters comes an extensive set of endnotes that offer additional reflections and also references to texts touching upon the current theme that could not be included in the main text. In this way the reader is given the opportunity to delve more deeply into topics of interest.

2

PSYCHOANALYSIS AS PRAXIS:
A PERSONAL VIEW

To reach an understanding of any obstacles to the psycho-analyst's professional development a point of reference is needed that may provide some notion of the values inherent in good analytical work. When analysts attempt to define such values they are often confronted with enumerations of such qualities or favorable dispositions that the good clinician must possess and/or acquire. The average list of such dispositions usually contains elements such as: a capacity for introspection; a capacity for identification; a capacity for empathy; a capacity for self-analysis; insight into their own weaknesses, limitations, and blind spots; that they regard analysis as something unique; integrity; maturity, with an emphasis on an integrated personality; emotional warmth; a capacity for self-discipline (from van der Leeuw 1962; see also Calef 1972:41–42; Grinberg 1989; Joseph 1978:383; Olinick et al. 1973). Still, there is something about this catalogue of desirable characteristics that misses the mark altogether.

Every attempt at a codification of good and sought-for qualities appears to conclude in a rather commonsensical outlook which, when all is said and done, really doesn't convey much. To some extent this may be a question of stylistic limitation, but I am inclined to believe that we are dealing here with a difficulty that is internal to the thing itself: *the good cannot be addressed with abstract formulations, it can only be practiced.*[1] The good is thus not a substance available for analyses and definitions. I therefore suggest that we take it for granted that the practice of psychoanalysis requires a certain minimum of competence, but that we invest our energies into formulating as good a description as possible of the task to be performed. In that way, competence will remain implied in the activity the description attempts to depict. This is not to say that this would be an easier task to perform than the construction of a catalogue of virtues—and let me say something about why I think this is so.

It is usually maintained that psychoanalysis is a method of treatment. That is indeed the way society and the general public judge it, and such is surely also the view of the future analysand as he or she concludes that now something must come about that will make life change for the better. On such a superordinate level psychoanalysis is not only an activity aiming at the removal of suffering and the liberation of creative forces—making people better equipped for envisaging and striving for a good life—but also a corrective measure to put right what for one reason or another has taken a deviant course.

I am quite sure that most analysts would agree with such a description. But on a more intimate level, it would most probably not be these purposes that they call upon to explain why they choose to spend such a large part of their lives in the pursuit of an activity that really doesn't resemble anything else. More probably, they would say (or think): "I do it because there is really nothing else I'd rather spend my time doing."

To those involved—analysand and analyst—analytic work is closest to what Aristotle calls a *praxis*, a self-fulfilling life activity. Once it is under way, analytic practice is its own incentive and its aims lie in the exercise itself. This is possibly what enables psychoanalysis to resist so perseveringly the most ambitious and well-intentioned attempts at defining it from the "outside." It has been an irritating fact to its critics and at times an embarrassment to its defenders that the deeper aspects of the psychoanalytic experience may perhaps be understood only through intimate acquaintance with its practice. In other words, we can only know what psychoanalysis is in the same way that we know what it is to be a human being. We know because we live—not necessarily with the best of experiences—but with experiences. We have our theories about the meaning of a good life only because we take part in it. The same goes for the application of the analytic method: "good technique" cannot really be understood other than as the analytic method when it proceeds in accordance with its intended pathways. To know really deep down what this "intended way" entails, one must have taken part in the psychoanalytic experience itself.

DIALOGICAL INTERPRETING

During the last ten to twenty years a model for reflection upon the analytic relationship has come to the fore that often is referred to as an "intersubjective" view. I believe that essentially, the issue of intersubjectivity does not have to do with theoretical preferences, nor does it primarily have to do with new clinical procedures, in the sense that Kleinian theory and technique once might have been a deviation from classical psychoanalysis. I would rather say that intersubjectivity is an attitude and a form of self-understanding, the greatest import of which has to do with how it brings forth aspects of analytic work that most probably have been present with all gifted psychoanalysts—regardless of theoretical inclination— for as long as our practice has been in existence. If that indeed is the case, then intersubjectivity—just like transference or defense— should have been regarded as an ineluctable dimension of the psychoanalytic experience and as such it is "eternal."[2]

The intersubjective model is founded on the conviction that psychoanalytic experience rests upon the unique human encounter. This also includes the belief that such an encounter can never be guided by supposed scientific knowledge, wherein the analysand is objectivated. In accordance with this, it is impossible to fall back on technical procedures and the reductionistic belief that there is an unconscious content lying in wait to be uncovered. Rather than conceiving of it in static terms, that is, as the correspondence between manifest (conscious) and unconscious representations, truth is seen as something always *on its way*, not a thing to possess, but a process embedded in the intersubjective dialectic of interpreting.[3]

Communication, Transference, and Countertransference

Freud wrote that "[i]t is a very remarkable thing that the *Ucs.* of one human being can react upon that of another, without passing through the *Cs.* This deserves closer investigation, [. . .] but, descriptively speaking, the fact is uncontestable" (Freud 1915:194). How shall we imagine that the unconscious communication Freud spoke of comes to pass, and what is characteristic of psychoanalytic interpreting?

To attempt an answer to these questions, I would first want to point out what I see as the prerequisite for analytic interpreting: an intersubjective structure I designate as a *matrix of communication*.[4] To be in the world is to be with others, a circumstance that makes our world a shared one. Man lives his presence in the world in an understanding and competent manner. Consequently, in the shared world of the matrix, we know, for the most part, *how* to go about things, even though this knowing is not always available to us in such a manner that we are able to explain *why* we do things the way we do. But our understanding is sufficient for us to live and survive—in our families, in the company of friends, and in our professions.

The experience that best lends itself to reflection on the existence of a matrix of communication is perhaps the first relation between the parent and the newborn child. The reciprocal attunement to the Being of the Other that shows in the adult's keenness in perceiving the child's needs and integrating them within a meaningful context and, equally, in the child's obvious sensitivity to the parent's moods, are living signs of the fundamental presence of a matrix of communication. From the point of view of standard psychoanalytic concepts, the matrix is situated at the level of the unconscious. Apart from its being the level of our competent "know-how" in living, it forms the basis for our utterances. That is to say that at the locus of the matrix a pristine psychic meaning is engendered, establishing a mutually embraced foundation of understanding that makes it possible for what I say to be received by my fellow human being as something intelligible.

The matrix of communication pertaining to the analytical situation has specific characteristics, which, of course, is due to its aim of establishing a field in which the analysand's transference is allowed to unfold. Transference is a two-sided phenomenon. In its most prominent aspect it stands out as the analysand's observable ways of construing the analyst as his object—not least how he creates a system of fantasies concerning the analyst's desire and what the analyst may want of him. Here we find that well-known spectrum of love and hate that in an almost uncanny way seems to awaken in practically every psychoanalytic treatment.

But these expressions of love and hate are merely the surface manifestations of the transference, for the analysand's passionate preoccupation with the person of the analyst is expressive of a veiled dimension that we could identify as the analysand's destiny. A person's destiny (i.e., that at once blind and omniscient unconscious life theme that takes hold and refuses to let go its grip, despite our efforts at interpreting and understanding, making amends or running away) is individual and private. Its way of action is repetition. We can say with full certainty that it was the unrelenting return of the same that drove the analysand to seek help when all other attempts had been futile.

I believe it is correct to claim that the form of psychoanalytical self-understanding mentioned above under the rubric of intersubjectivity is an extension of a movement that arose during the fifties, when a group of English psychoanalysts initiated a productive discussion concerning the interaction between the analysand's transference and that form of participation on the analyst's part that is usually called "countertransference." Originally, the term "counter-transference" was coined by Freud to designate the analyst's unproductive or harmful actions caused by his unconscious reactions to the analysand's transference. The phenomenon was at that time regarded as the expression of the analyst's "blind spots," a sort of flaw in the instrument of analytic listening that it was hoped could be done away with through the further analysis of the analyst: "Back to the couch!"

These English clinicians extended the conditions of analytic listening by presenting a wider definition of countertransference, which now also would include the affect-laden inner processes the analyst could experience in response to the analysand's unconscious communication. In this way, countertransference became an instrument for the discernment of something yet unarticulated within the analysand, which, for one reason or another, had not managed to find an adequate form of expression. What remains problematic for me with this conception, however, is that it preserves a view of the relationship between analyst and analysand that is analogous to that between a subject and its object: the analyst is expected to make interpretations of unconscious content residing in the analysand, even though these temporarily might have been deposited within his own being.

In line with the conception proposed here, that the partners in the analytic relationship are involved in an intersubjective matrix of communication, I would say that the term "countertransference" does not fit well with the phenomenon that these English analysts wished to designate. I would suggest that we rather maintain Freud's original definitions and consequently reserve the concept of countertransference for those aspects of the analyst's stance with regard to the analysand that are occasioned by unanalyzed, disturbing, or even destructive aspects of his own personality.

From an intersubjective point of view, the analyst's affective reactions in interaction with the analysand are an obvious and inevitable aspect of the analyst's participation in the matrix, and surely nothing that would "go counterwise," as if *against* the process. Instead of countertransference, we should more accurately speak of the analyst's *co*transference. And—let it be noted—the cotransference is just as idiosyncratic and founded upon an individual and mainly unconscious destiny as is the analysand's transference.[5]

A vital aspect of the psychoanalyst's competence is his ability to attune his listening to that part of the matrix that borders on the analysand's wholly private world. The vital difference between the respective positions of analyst and analysand lies in the implicit agreement that the analysand's transference will set the theme for the interpreting, while the analyst's cotransference will function as a disciplined instrument for monitoring this process. The analyst makes his presence available as a sheltering container of the analysand's destiny. The discipline involved in this has to do with the analyst taking upon himself the task of defending the specific integrity of the analytic situation, that is, the arrangements in time and space making it possible for such a relation to evolve (more concerning the analytic setting in Chapter 4).

The Matrix of Transference

Analytic interpreting grows from the interplay between transference and cotransference, as contained within the boundaries of the matrix of communication. At the outset of an analytic enterprise, the communicative matrix may not differ greatly from other matrices underlying our social relationships. But, depending on the individual and shared qualifications of both participants, a transition slowly takes place, as the analyst acquaints himself with the world in which the analysand moves and unfolds his being. Also the opposite will occur, and at this level, where "the *Ucs.* of one human being can react upon that of another, without passing through the *Cs.*," it is perhaps most appropriate to say that the kind of communication in question evolves through the fact that analyst and analysand *get to know each other*. And getting to know someone is a process that in its most important aspects takes place outside of either of the participants' knowl-

edge and capacity for control. In fact, it is the opposite of knowledge and more a question of *being*.

Transference certainly does have something unreal about it,
like a fictitious state saturated with fantastic themes, dependency
feelings, and desires of a kind we otherwise seldom let ourselves
come in touch with. But putting too great an emphasis on its illu-
sory character will obscure the fact that within its boundaries a
degree of urgency reveals itself, which can only be accounted for
as the manifestation of the desire and psychic reality of both participants. In other words, transference—and cotransference—are
underpinned by the strictest earnestness, with a presence and an
intimacy that will not shy away from any of the passions. In its
reign, each party is given the possibility of coming closest to his
own essence, while at the same time deeply affected by the being
of the Other.

And with that, the matrix of communication has become a
matrix of transference. This is the core of psychoanalytic intersubjectivity, and the playground for a shared life. The psychic
reality in force here can never be observed, but only interpreted.
The matrix of transference is a common affective field, where the
respective positions of the participants are permeable to each
other, which is why, experientially, they cannot always be distinguished. To me, this permeability is the most likely basis for
explaining Freud's observation concerning the unconscious communication between two subjects.

The matrix makes it possible to grasp, for example, the clinically observable fact that transference is never pure fiction, but
instead readily crystallizes around existing traits in the analyst.
This will also shed some light on how—in instances when the
transference will hold back for a while—the analysand may have
very poignant observations concerning the analyst's person to
report. Or those remarkable "telepathic" phenomena that will
manifest themselves in how analyst and analysand on one and
the same night may have dreams that thematically complement
each other. Or that the analysand, in his associations, displays
veritable insights into the analyst's present situation, which

could be anything ranging from practical concerns occupying him to details having to do with his family relations.

Vignette

To exemplify the above considerations I would like to interfoliate with an extract from the reconstruction of the analytical dialogue between me and a female analysand, whom I here call Eve.

Eve: I have a gastric flu today. I threw up all night and have diarrhea, so I may suddenly have to run for the toilet during our session.

Analyst: Mmm.

Eve: I was wondering whether I should come or not, but I had so many thoughts after yesterday's session that I felt I must. I thought that maybe there was a risk of me transmitting the infection to you and everyone else coming here today.

A: Mmm.

Eve: After the session yesterday I kept on thinking about the curiosity I had about my parents' sex life. During lunch at my job I sat down with a couple of colleagues engaged in some discussion and I just asked what they were talking about, even though I realized that perhaps they didn't want to be disturbed. They were talking about that new managerial position that has been advertised.

A: Mmm.

Eve: And then of course I thought about what you brought up about there perhaps being some kind of erotic tension in relation to you. I had really thought that, well, this must have been cleared up by now—but of course that's not the way it is. [Silence] It feels like you're distraught, as if you're preoccupied with something else . . . [Silence] I really think I'm going to apply for that manager job. It's a chance in a million.

A: I thought that perhaps it's important to you to come today despite your misgivings about possibly infecting me because it's important to show me that you're not grown up, but a shitty little brat.[6]

Eve: Yes, that could be. What you said about eventual sexual tension actually worried me yesterday. I was thinking about that when I left here. It's funny, shitty brat doesn't sound terrible at all and not insulting either. [Silence] If I were to get that job, then I wouldn't be a shitty brat anymore . . .

A: No, and maybe you would find yourself to be on the same level as I, so that you might become a possible partner or object for my sexual interest.

Eve: That's true. I remember when I was thirteen and waiting for my periods to start, like I told you yesterday. I was on a trip with my father and at one time a trickle of blood actually came and I reacted with immediate joy. But . . . it came from my anus. They had such rough toilet paper at that place.

A: Just shit, then. I guess it would have been a great thing for you to have your first menstruation while you were alone with your father.

Eve: Oh, yes! I was so disappointed. It came somewhat later, when I was at some church camp. Totally wrong . . . [Silence] There was something special with my father. And he could laugh like my mother never could. He joked and played on words. He often made me laugh, too.

During our session last Friday, by the way, you and I were joking together and I felt I had to hold back, because I felt like it was indecent. Later the same day when I was thinking about what you had said I had to laugh aloud several times. But to laugh here with you . . . it's almost as if there were something erotic in it. [Silence] No, my mother wasn't much to laugh with. But she would take care of me if I was sick . . . like today, for example. I remember the feeling when I was lying on the sofa listening to her bustling about in the kitchen. And then she would bring the milk bottle. I had it for a long time, until I was five I think. Maybe that was the same time as when my sister and I got our own rooms and I was alone by myself.

A: A nursing bottle?

Eve: Yes, and there was such a fuss about it. Had it been standing for too long and there was a film on it, I would just reject it. I guess that's the room that became the first secret room.

A: Mmm.

[Silence]

Eve: At that time my father was gone for six months. And when he came back it was as if he hadn't noticed at all that I'd grown. He was too preoccupied with his depression. I actually don't believe that he noticed how I was developing into a woman later when I was thirteen.

A: It sounds a bit like wishful thinking on your part that he would be so preoccupied with his depression that he wouldn't notice that you were growing to be a woman.

Eve: So that it wouldn't become dangerous and sexual.

A: Maybe that's why you preferred to imagine that I was distraught and busy with something else earlier during this session.

Eve: Yes, and that I'd rather be a shitty brat than confess to being a grown-up woman in this room together with you, with all the emotions that could bring. . . .

This vignette was not chosen with the aim of promoting any particular thesis or to establish any definite fact concerning the psychoanalytic experience. One could very well object that in my example the analytical dialogue is represented in a way that makes it appear like something that flows easily and the analyst as the one who knows. It is quite clear that during a session such as this I do not have to use all my available energy to maintain my capacity for thought, or my interest and benevolence, something that is often called upon during periods of so-called negative transference and that is part of the competence the analyst must possess. It is also quite apparent that the communication here is concentrated upon interpreting, and for that reason the decisive actions are mainly of a purely verbal nature. In other clinical situations the most essential thing may be that the analyst merely be present in such a way that the analysand is helped in experiencing that she exists at all and that this can be something good.

There are no "typical" sessions; if there is anything typical of the psychoanalytic experience it is the uncertainty that both parties, for the most part, are immersed in. Still, this vignette is instructive. I chose it because at the time this session took place, it felt good, like a "successful" session in that elusive sense suggested above: it felt good because it developed precisely according to the kind of psychoanalysis that I try to practice. It is instructive because it offers a clear picture of how the analysand's current relation to the analyst in the transference intertwines with the destiny codified through the life history that can be reconstructed.

Eve presents a fantasy, which, according to received analytical lines of thought, could easily lend itself to interpretations in aggressive terms—for example, as the sign of a desire to drench the analyst in feces and infect all the siblings. Such a possibility did occur to me, but it did not feel right to say anything about it just then. Something—and I cannot say what—was telling me that in this instance something else was at stake and therefore I chose to follow one of the most important rules of the analytical attitude: wait and see.

Eve's comment that I seemed to be preoccupied with something other than her was most probably what triggered my first intervention. It was a way of responding to an existentially demanding situation in which Eve started to feel abandoned. I believe I wished to show her that I was there. At the same time I entertained the hope of stopping this fantasy of my absence from growing stronger, as it might disturb other and more promising threads of thought. Thus I said to Eve that more than anything else she wished to present herself as a shitty brat. With hindsight, a daring attempt, I think, since it could be misunderstood, and the risk that Eve would perceive my comment as condescending or critical was not negligible. But my direct appeal to the little shitty brat included a clear intention of conveying not only the warmth I felt for the child who had come to me in all its literal shittiness, but also the respect I felt for Eve's struggle to be a grown-up woman. In this way, I think, she could feel that "shitty brat" need be neither appalling nor insulting.

The "shitty brat" intervention was an experiment that turned out to be decisive for the rest of the session. I made Eve focus on an issue that at the beginning of the session existed in her scope only as one of several possible associative threads. With my intervention I suggested: "Let's try this thought out for a moment and see if it holds." I took a risk in demanding that Eve look at the situation from that point of view. Her confirmation of my hunch did not so much lie in her saying, "Yes, that could be it," but rather in the fact that she offered a whole row of new associations fitting the theme. Her associations became somewhat of a reward system, encouraging me to continue along the chosen path and even to persevere when other paths do turn up—as, for example, when she started talking about the mother, the nursing bottle, and the secret room.

With my "shitty brat" intervention I was the one to decide what theme was to be the most central and productive just then, thus contributing to how the rest of the session was to develop. And I did apparently manage to appeal to something within her that at that moment was in harmony both with the chosen theme and her curiosity and willingness to make new discoveries. Not that I could know what was going to happen if I did this or that, but Eve's associations were in reply to something I was responsible for having brought into the discussion. What was truly rewarding in this interaction was that the ensuing course of events would uncover things that neither of us was aware of as I formulated my hunch.

With Evenly Suspended Attention

When it is most genuine, psychoanalytic interpreting picks up its vital thrust from the shared world of the matrix. The competence of the psychoanalyst rests to a large extent upon his attentiveness when it comes to the variations and modulations in the analysand's transference, together with the capacity to maintain the singular mix belonging to the analytic situation of curiosity, playfulness, and deepest seriousness. The analyst's foremost "method" for listening in this respect is that procedure Freud called *gleichschwebende Aufmerksamkeit*—evenly suspended attention (Freud 1912:111): "to avoid so far as possible reflection and the construction of conscious expectations, not to try to fix anything that he heard particularly in his memory, and by these means to catch the drift of the patient's unconscious with his own unconscious" (Freud 1923a:239). Evenly suspended attention is a kind of meditative heed, where the analyst strives to relinquish the ego's demand for comprehension and context, and instead provides a response to something beyond the immediate sense inherent in the analysand's speech.

To follow the wording of Freud's expression, we might say that *evenly* indicates an equal interest in what is high and what is low, for the inner and the outer, for the good and the bad. *Suspended* suggests a lack of allegiance to determined lines of thought and preset models of interpretation; furthermore, it implies the absence of moral or judgmental engagements. *Attention*, finally, leads us to think in terms of interest, curiosity, love, faith, and responsibility.

There is one guiding rule for evenly suspended listening, namely that the analyst maintain the most keen vigilance with regard to what in every moment is most urgent in the analysand's relation to his destiny. In that sense, the ethos of psychoanalysis may at times seem to collide brutally with our everyday ethic of care. It is, of course, true that a kind of superordinate ethic of care does hover over the resolution of the analytical attitude never to leave the analysand abandoned with his affects and his situation, but instead—as far as this is possible—to remain with the analysand and help him identify his condition. But the primary task of the analyst is not to be a good and benevolent fellow being. His function is to promote understanding and change, and when that purpose is given precedence the merciful impulse to offer sustenance, consolation, or guidance will have to stand back (just like the impulse to judge, condemn, or punish, which at times may appear on the analysand's agenda).

In my experience, analytical interventions are *actions* that do not necessarily pertain to an identified object. Listening with evenly suspended attention to the unconscious communication of the matrix is not the same as turning one's attention to a presupposed latent content in the analysand's utterances, and the relationship between analyst and analysand is not a relationship between the analyst's ego and the analysand as its object of knowledge. Instead, analytic interpreting is an exposition of an experience that evolves as analyst and analysand allow themselves to be engaged in the intersubjective dimension of the matrix, where the one is part of the other's world, and vice versa.

For that reason, the analyst turns his capacity for listening *inward*, toward that part of his own psychic reality that in the shared world of the matrix has blended with that of the analysand. In the vignette above, Eve's presence within the matrix of transference lent to her utterances and fantasies—despite whatever else they may concern—the capacity to convey messages about the analytical situation and her relation to me. On the basis of this shared ground it was also possible for me to work *within* the transference, as I grasped themes pertaining partly to the present and partly to predecessors in Eve's life around which similar themes had once revolved. To the same extent, that very presence gave her the possibilty of validating my interventions. The legitimacy of analytic interpreting—and its value as truth— rests wholly upon the shared presence in the matrix of transference. Here lies the good basis for analytical work that makes it possible, *with the precision of heedful action*, to convey something of determined importance to the analysand's current relation to his destiny.

Analytic interventions are part of an overarching and comprehensive movement, where, strictly speaking, there is never a question of interpretations, but a constant interpreting-in-process that is not limited to one or the other of the participants, and that cannot be tied to individual interventions. *Analytic interpreting consists in the dialogical course of events as such.* Everything happening in the room—from the analysand's productions to the analyst's responses—is part of this process, where the manifest transference itself is the interpreting of a destiny.[7]

The Process of Clinical Reflection

An intersubjective view of psychoanalytic interpreting will entail a somewhat unorthodox way of looking at the place and function of clinical reflection. It is no longer a question of the analyst listening to what the analysand says and then distancing himself from the situation to reflect and reaching an understanding that he then may convey in the form of an interpretation. There are no fundamental obstacles to a remote reflection upon the elements of the analytic dialogue. This can be done between sessions, in discussions with colleagues, in secluded contemplation, or when writing a text. But during the sessions, analyst and analysand are engaged in the business of life itself, and their respective contributions to the interpreting dialogue are parts of the same process of reflection. Like interpreting, reflection evolves as an integral part of the course of events.

Let us assume the existence of something we might call the analyst's "clinical hypothesis." Let us further assume that the clinical hypothesis is a sort of equivalent to the hypothesis a scientist would formulate and then set about to test by conducting an experiment. But, in contradistinction to the conditions obtaining in such an ideal case, the analyst's clinical hypothesis can only be assumed. In the actual clinical situation, the hypothesis exists merely as an anticipation, and only conceptually can it be separated from the experiment itself. The formulation of the hypothesis and the experimentation unfold in one and the same movement.

With my "shitty brat" intervention in the vignette above I gathered not only from my impression of the session's initial interchange with its variegated directions and entrances, but also from the previous day's work. I offered a hypothesis concerning what at that precise moment might have been of the most central importance in Eve's mind and that despite her stomach affliction she chose to come to her session. My intervention was based upon a premonition carrying the implicit clinical hypothesis concerning Eve's current predicament, her intentions, needs, and desires. (In that real situation I am allowed to learn something about my own unconscious thoughts by translating them into some kind of intervention. Only in connection with the reconstruction of this clinical example has it been possible for me to ponder what thoughts my premonitions might have been based upon.)

As to the analyst, the fact that he has something meaningful to say is the empirical criterion that understanding is at hand, even when he perhaps has not fully grasped the sense of what the analysand has said so that he might not be able to make an interpretation of what he has just heard. The analyst's meaningful intervention is the heedful response to their common situation. This activity on the part of the analyst is very close to free associating, a way of relating to clinical reality that perhaps is even more indispensable in his case—for how else is the analysand to be expected to develop an acquaintance with it?

The analyst's anticipation projects toward the future a meaning residing in his understanding. This is not to be taken to be a "plan" of the ego, but rather a trace, along which future interpreting may come to unfold. But, of this nothing is known as long as no words have been uttered. The analyst gains insight into his participation in the unconscious communication of the matrix by transforming his anticipations into some form of intervention. According to the motto, "I know not what I think before I have spoken," understanding comes to be realized as knowledge only through the interpreting dialogue.

The same pertains to the analysand's utterances, which, even if it may take time before this becomes evident to any of the participants, are always directed by the intention of coming to speech about that which is existentially most urgent. Eve gets to know something about her own unconscious processes and her relation to her destiny through the responses she receives in the form of the continued interpreting dialogue.

Hope and Faith

The interpreting dialogue requires time. This is one of the main reasons analysand and analyst have to meet as many as five times a week during the course of several years—not only because it takes time for two people to get to know each other, but because interpreting takes its own, often unpredictable, ways and the turns must be repeated numerous times—worked through, says Freud—for insight and permanent change to occur. To the analysand, this may turn out to be a demanding experience, as he must be able to entertain so much hope that he can wait through the great amount of time it takes. Sometimes this resource is lacking, and then it will be up to the analyst to support the necessary hope. In a tacit agreement that is difficult to unravel, the analysand is then given the possibility of abandoning himself to his lack of hope, while in the meantime the analyst keeps harboring a light, of which it may become clear only much later that that keepsake was in fact the analysand's very own.

For his own part, the analyst has to deal with another kind of hope, which I call "faith in the Other."[8] Fundamentally, the Other is always beyond the reach of my knowledge, my fantasies, or my wish to objectify him. Faith in the Other is the sustained hope that I, despite his unrelenting unavailability, will meet him in his subjectivity. Faith shapes a horizon of anticipation that in turn establishes a specific kind of analytical space, making it possible for the analyst to *await* the analysand. This kind of faith will in no way override or do away with the fundamental mystery of the Other, but it does offer a way of living without knowledge.

Faith in the Other is vital for the psychoanalyst's capacity to genuinely uphold his interest and his presence within the matrix of transference. The characteristic mark of evenly suspended attention is the tolerance for the uncertainty and lack of knowing that it exercises. Before all else it is an attitude of *expectancy* founded in the faith that truth and more understanding are on their way.

Awaiting the Other may possibly be taken to be a passive stance. Nothing could be more erroneous, but that does not mean that expectancy can be designated as a form of activity. Awaiting the Other is the ethical mark of evenly suspended attention; it is the postponement of articulated reflection, thematization, and objectivation. It is being rather than doing, knowing than knowledging. It is *being capable.*

It belongs to the ethos of psychoanalysis to respect the uniqueness of the analysand—which means that the analyst will strive to persevere in ignorance rather than to arrive at quick conclusions, to listen rather than to make assertions. Essentially, this is an ethic respectful of the fact that neither the Other nor the unconscious can be mastered by knowledge. Therefore I consider faith in the Other to be integral to the analytical attitude and to the analyst's ethical commitment with regard to the analysand.

When the analyst's faith in the Other vacillates and is disturbed, something very decisive occurs, which I believe may be observed in such instances when analytical interpreting turns into the "making of interpretations." As a fact belonging to the tragic dimension of psychoanalytic experience, we do at times turn from talking *with* the analysand to talking *to* him, and the process remains sensitive to this kind of deviance from the analyst's commitment.

One could in this connection speak of an *ethical failure*—not unlike how American self-psychologists speak of "empathic failure." Ethical failure has to do with the analyst's inevitable shortcomings. In themselves they are unavoidable, but when we manage to identify them together with the analysand, they may serve as a source for new insights and widened experience for both participants.

The Faithfulness of Truth

This is an issue bordering upon the dimension of truth in psychoanalytic interpreting. Wilfred Bion writes: "Worse than being right or wrong is the failure of an interpretation to be significant, though to be significant is not enough; it merely ensures that it exists. It must also be true" (1970:79). What, then—from the point of view of communication and interpreting developed here—can be said concerning analytic work and its relation to truth?

First of all, I would like to suggest that "significance," in the sense Bion uses the word here, is a quality wholly independent of the participants' psychological "understanding" or "empathy." Significance has rather to do with a quality belonging to their mutual responses, confirming those areas of their matrix of communication where they meaningfully affect each other.

When we then turn to that quality Bion refers to as "truth," we may start out by saying that truth is that which appears through the interpreting dialogue, not as an item to be possessed, but something always *on its way*—like the interpreting course of events itself. And, if it really is true that truth resides in a course of events rather than in individual utterances, the particular intervention can neither be true nor false; it can only be part of a context in motion toward or away from truth. The individual elements of the interpreting dialogue must not univocally point in the same direction, or be in accord with and corroborate each other for it to be possible to regard them as true in this sense.

But have we not, with this, moved to grounds where in fact it is no longer possible to speak at all of truth—at least as long as we stick to a classical definition that says that truth resides in the adequation between a thought and its object—or, when it comes to psychoanalysis, the adequation between an utterance and its unconscious correlate (which could be a fantasy or an idea)? Rather than "truth," we might do better speaking of "faithfulness."

The possibility for faithfulness makes its appearance at the interval between understanding and interpreting. The only guarantee that saying is on its way to truth is in the resolve of interpreting to be faithful to the meaning that has been handed over in the form of an anticipation. Here no promises can be made, for any interpreting can be questioned and every story retold from a new angle. But, in the psychoanalytic experience, resolve in faithfulness is most probably the closest we can come to any assurance that truth is likely to be on its way.

ON THEORETICAL WORK

Theories have, by their very nature, to be abandoned.
—N. Symington 1986:19

When one reads reconstructions of the analytic dialogue it is striking how the theoretical language of psychoanalysis is almost totally absent. Instead, the communication within the analytic relationship rests upon a developed and sophisticated version of commonsense psychology. By commonsense psychology I mean such knowing[9] that we are all in possession of for our conventional reflection concerning ourselves and others. Our commonsense psychology is not only part of the competence with which we deal with the world and our interpersonal relationships, but is also part of our capacity—in the form of both personal and social narratives—to convey in words our own and other persons' mental states in terms of experiences, feelings, needs, and motives. The interpreting interventions of the dialogic interaction between analysand and analyst are formulated in the language of commonsense psychology, making it possible for the analysand—who most often will lack any theoretical knowledge—to recognize his own experience through introspection, insight, or identification, and reflect upon it with new associations.

Thus, listening to the unconscious communication of the transferential relationship with evenly suspended attention presupposes that in some important sense we have left theoretical knowledge behind. Theory is not a catalogue of insights, near at hand, to be carried along when encountering the analysand. It is not a faithful image of what takes place in the communicative matrix of the analytical situation. Instead, theory is a construction of a very special kind.

If, as analysts, we suppose that by dint of our theories we are in possession of an instrument for discerning the unconscious preconditions for the objects or fantasies manifesting themselves in the analysand's transference, we are, in my view, mistaken—for to interpret is to follow the movements of the transferential relationship while listening to one's own presence rather than to knowledge. Here, however, the culture transmitted within the psychoanalytic training system tends to pass this misconception on. Thus psychoanalysis runs the risk of not only befuddling its own self-understanding, but also of undermining its immanent ethic.

To this ethic belongs, as we saw above, endurance of the fact that we can have no knowledge, either of the Other or of the unconscious. In itself, theory does no more than allow us to perceive the mechanics of an objectivated psychological machinery, and therefore it tends to split our perception between what we are actually experiencing in the analytic encounter and what it demands that we see. To come in touch with clinical experience, theoretical knowledge must be transformed into competence. That is to say, for it to become fully fit for use in the transference relationship it must be incorporated within the very being of the psychoanalyst—it must "become flesh." This comes about through a specific form of achievement that I shall simply call *theoretical work*.

Theoretical work is a variegated process that forms an experience in its own right, which, like all experience, will affect those who partake in it. I regard theoretical work as a spiritual exercise, a form of meditation in preparation for a return to the analytic encounter with new knowing and an altered readiness for hearing, seeing, and discovering. For the results of that work to deserve credence, the theorist's deepest insights and convictions as to what it is to be a human being and a psychoanalyst must be engaged.[10]

Three Levels of Psychoanalytic Knowing

Whenever psychoanalytic knowing is referred to, most people probably have in mind what is called clinical theory. Not only is clinical theory most often the façade that psychoanalysis turns toward the surrounding world as the part of the analytic experience that is most easy to convey to outsiders, but, more important, it is also a codified body of knowledge that every psychoanalyst, at least to some extent, has made his own and has identified with.

The way it is understood here, though, psychoanalytic knowing comprises three distinct levels, of which the experience that unfolds in the clinical encounter between analyst and analysand comes first and is most fundamental. This aspect of the analyst's knowing consists not only of his experience of conducting analytic work, but also of himself having once been an analysand. The language employed in the clinical situation is that of common-sense psychology.

The second level of analytic knowing is clinical theory, which on one side is flanked by the knowing of clinical experience, and on the other by metapsychology, which constitutes the third level. Theoretical work is executed within all three, albeit in a different key and with differing aims. The theoretical work related to the level of clinical experience I call *assimilation*; clinical theory and metapsychology are mutually dependent and the work belonging to these levels I call *construction*. In addition, all three levels of theoretical work presuppose a process I call *deconstruction*.

Construction: Clinical Theory

By nature, commonsense psychology is "untamed" and "wild" in the sense that it stays close to the commonplace knowledge belonging to general ideology and easily corrupts unless regulated by disciplined theoretical work. In its ideological form, commonsense knowledge serves to corroborate what we already know and, in the long run, it can only give support to our prejudices, existing relations of power, and so forth. To take an example: the most salient aspects of ideological knowing in psychoanalytic thinking are its notions concerning normality, maturity, and pathology. It may be inevitable that psychoanalysis must busy itself with these categories, but the values invested in such discourse can nevertheless only be ideological in nature.

It is important that one appreciate the necessary distance between commonsense understanding in the clinical situation and theoretical knowledge—between what can be described and what cannot be observed—for it to be possible to question the former with the help of the latter. Precisely this would be one of the most important tasks for a clinical theory.[11]

There is noticeable pressure directed at psychoanalytic knowing arising *inter alia* from the deep wish of analysands that we give them love rather than analyze them, as well as from an environment that finds it difficult to accept that so much time and so many resources are bestowed upon individual persons in a praxis that has obvious difficulties in accounting for its results (which in turn has to do with the fact that its true merits can only be appreciated through personal experience). Together, these demands that psychoanalysis should always be something else— cheaper, more expedient, and more comprehensible, while at the same time preaching an unmistakable message of love—form a threat to the integrity of both its practice and its knowing. One important way of safeguarding this integrity is theoretical work, which is a sort of monitoring in which our commonsense psychology is repaired and refurbished when it proves to be inadequate or threatens to water down to ideology.

A not uncommon conception of the interplay between theory and practice holds that psychoanalytic theory is a language for describing and/or explaining certain aspects of the world of psychoanalytic experience. So, for example, one can come across the view that theory can provide a phenomenology of the unconscious phantasmatic world (see, for example, Steiner 1985:41), and, by implication, that when properly informed theoretically, the analyst would have privileged access to the analysand's unconscious. And, from a certain point of view it is, of course, correct to say that clinical theory is that part of analytic knowing that is used to better understand and deepen our description of clinical experience. It would contribute to this by offering acceptable explanations. To that extent it would be part of a relatively uncomplicated hermeneutical dialectic between explanations and enhanced understanding. But that still misses the core issue, for theory is not the language of clinical experience and should not first-handedly be taken as an attempt to provide the best possible interpretation of the clinical encounter with the analysand.

It seems, however, that psychoanalytic theory really has nothing more to offer but speculation and fiction, albeit a very controlled speculation taking as its starting point the experience of the clinical situation. This may sound like a shortcoming, but should rather be seen as a possibility for freedom from the power of unreflected habit and its strong affinity with ideological knowledge.

We would most probably be more realistic if instead we were to regard theory as a language for *opening up* the world. The primary function of psychoanalytic theory—clinical theory *and* metapsychology—would then be to inform the analyst's capacity for listening and responding to the analysand, rather than to provide a map of reality.

The above-mentioned freedom from the power of habit is connected with how theoretical work deconstructs commonsense knowing (just as it does with existing theories; see below). Commonsense psychology, as was intimated earlier, is characterized by being accessible to introspection and identification. This is the language in which we all move in our everyday reflection upon our experience. The deconstructive moment of theoretical work operates by replacing the categories of this common language with a structure of abstract and systematically interrelated concepts that, due to their deliberate nature, do not allow for direct empathic appropriation as the former categories do. An example of this would be how words like "person" or "mother" in theory may be represented by the concept of "object." Precisely because it is a fiction contrived to speak about an assumed *psychic reality* (individual or intersubjectively shared) underlying the psychological realm (and distinct from it), the language of clinical theory itself is only seemingly psychological.

In my view, if no deconstruction of the commonsensical and its ideological elements has taken place, insufficient theoretical work has been carried out and no true theory has been engendered. However, when theoretical work has been sufficiently completed, the constructed concepts of clinical theory will form an independent object for thought, a separate reality at a remove from the realm of clinical experience and the commonsense language usually employed to speak of it.

One of the consequences of the distance between the language of theory and the language of experience is that theory, at least to begin with, must be appropriated by purely intellectual means. Only thereafter—and gradually—can a work of assimilation and a return to commonsense knowing be embarked upon.

Theoretical work never takes place in a void, but always within a tradition, that is, against a background of formulated and assimilated theories as well as knowledge deriving from other disciplines. Were it not for the fact that existing theories in one way or another are experienced by some individual psychoanalysts as inadequate or lacking credibility, new theory would never be formulated. For that reason, theoretical work includes a preliminary critique of received theory in order to establish its struc-

ture and how it relates to, for example, the metaphysical foundations for one's own convictions. This form of deconstructive
work—which differs from the kind just discussed but which is
equally an integral part of constructive theoretical work—will sort
out those aspects of existing theory that can be deemed still valid
from those concepts and suppositions that appear to be incompatible with the structure slowly evolving in conjunction with
the present theoretical work.

In addition, there is something even more elusive, which has
to do with the capacity (or lack thereof) of the concepts to create
a sense of credibility as to their meaning content. As was mentioned, theoretical work seeks to elaborate a conceptual structure
adequate for speaking of the assumed psychic reality underlying
what we might call life's flow of psychologically available passions and dramas, especially as these appear in the transference
relationship of the analytic situation. The active theoretician's
personal experience of psychoanalytical practice is the ultimate
point of reference for the decision whether or not the concepts
forged have something meaningful to convey in this sense, despite their fictitious nature. This judgmental function—which is
founded upon a complex interaction taking place between moments of deconstruction, speculative creation, and the living presence of analytical experience—resides in refined unconscious
thought processes that seem to elude our introspective capacities.

Thus is engendered, in a labyrinthine process with many im-
passes and necessary failures, a separate theoretical object, a conceptual structure that must not be presumed to coincide or be
isomorphic with the psychic reality of which it purports to speak.
(Like Freud, I assume a realistic stance when it comes to the onto-
logical status of the unconscious.) Here we find concepts relating
to the analysand's expected intrapsychic contents, describing the
"inner world" of analysands, for example, in terms of objects and
the emotionally and affectively charged relations obtaining between
these in the form of complexes or unconscious fantasies.

On the basis of the concepts invented in theoretical work, some
kind of narrative presentation must be produced. For even if we,

in our minds, may be able to conceive of the theory in terms of pure structures, it most often takes some kind of narrative exposition to make it manageable as a form of knowledge.[12] Examples of this would be how most clinical theory is amalgamated with a developmental perspective—as in the theory of the Oedipus complex and its dissolution, the notion of an oscillating movement between the paranoid-schizoid and depressive positions, or the transformations of typical unconscious fantasies.

The introduction of narrative into the language of theory brings two consequences. Because the narrative form tends to borrow its matter from the language of commonsense psychology, which in this way steals back into theory again, it will on the one hand offer a new point of attack for the omnipresent tendency to ideological erosion. On the other hand, it will give rise to structurally conditioned demands regarding what a narrative presentation must include: for example, a trustworthy beginning.

In this way, clinical theory will have great affinity with the mythical dimension. Myth has the function of satisfying a desire that arises from the narrative structure itself, as can be recognized in Aristotle's well-known statement that every good plot must have a beginning, a middle, and an end. As the teller of, for example, a developmental history, the theorist is obliged to seek or create an origin for the plot of the story—say, in terms of the complexes or unconscious fantasies just mentioned—that he himself and those about him may have confidence in. Myths of that kind aim at speaking of the deepest wells of our existence while, at the same time, they serve the function of appeasing the theorist's appetite for context and narrative order.

Assimilation

Edward Glover describes the analyst's psychological knowing as "an exercise in imagination . . . imagination is the most economical of all instruments of research, often short-circuiting current modes of thought by the application of unconscious modes to the problem in hand" (1968:7). I would like to augment Glover's statement and say that fantasy characterizes psychoanalytical thinking from beginning to end. When, for example, Wilfred Bion describes how an analysand takes a part of the analyst into himself, as if sucking something out of him, and then expels it to have it deposited in a corner of the office (1958:65–67), this is a fantasy that Bion offers (or possibly shares with) the analysand on the basis of their joint experience in the transference relationship. Interpreting and the making of clinical descriptions demand work on the level of fantasy, and the same fantasy function has to be engaged in the construction of clinical theory.

Since it is a fantasy material, a theory is laden with the unconscious thought processes of the person who created it. As such, any theory is a symptom, an idiosyncratic interpretation, and a compromise formation. We may let ourselves be affected by Bion's sensitivity before his analysand, but we will surely lose something personally very important to us if—in our own work, theoretical or clinical—we take after (imitate) his fantasy concerning what once passed in his experience, as it is inert matter, a mere relic left behind by what was once intense fantasy work. Bion's clinical truth cannot be my or your truth. Likewise, those who in their practice assume the theory of another, choose to live in and by another person's symptomatic fantasy (see Roustang 1982:55–64). The implication here is, of course, that theory has to be continually reinvented.

The possibility lying open to us of welcoming a theory or rejecting it as incompatible with our most considered reflection has, first of all, to do with to what extent it may be verified through introspection (which, in this connection, I see as the balancing of whether the claims of the theory accord with our own experience) and through comparison with our more philosophical or metaphysical convictions concerning human existence. But even when, with the help of such an intellectual approach, we have found a theory to be valid and have taken it to heart, we must let it undergo a process of assimilation before it can come to good clinical use.

The work of assimilation has the function of making the analyst's commonsensical psychological knowing congruent, in part, with the inherent structure of the knowledge conveyed by the theory. The moment of deconstruction implied here resides in knowledge being *sublated* in a (Hegelian) dialectical sense, and this occurs as the theory is emptied of its fantastic and narrative forms while at the same time its meaningful gestalt or conceptual structure is preserved on the level of commonsensical psychological knowing (thus unconsciously).

While, on the one hand, assimilation is tantamount to deconstructing a material produced on the basis of fantasy, it is itself an exercise in tracing a web of thoughts and fancies issuing from the imaginative faculty of fantasy. Such a transformation may take place, for example, when we abandon ourselves before the theoretical text to the fecund inventiveness of intuition, as when memories of our own experiences and those of others are allowed to well up and be perceived in the light of theoretical knowledge. It can also happen during clinical discussions, in supervision, or in seminars, where theory is connected with the interaction between analysand and analyst. Another way for assimilation to take place might be the writing of a case report integrating a purely clinical description with some theoretical issue.

But more important than any of these "organized" forms of assimilation is the analyst's solitary encounter with theory. Years of acquaintance with psychoanalytic knowledge will gradually make the analyst forgetful of the impact that these theories once had. In all probability, though, few of us were ever spared from more or less excruciating bouts of hypochondria each time some new theory concerning psychosis, narcissism, perversion, or borderline states was to be learned. The working through—in solitary introspection and/or in analysis—that must be accomplished to digest the sometimes shocking effect that theory can have upon us, is to me a good illustration of how a process of assimilation may take place. And even when we do not make a detour into hypochondriacal anxiety, assimilation still demands that, to some extent, we retain a state of pristine naïveté allowing us to go beyond intellectual apprehension and be *affected* by the theory. Only when something like that happens is the faculty of imagination truly set in motion.

The work of assimilation establishes important links between our lived experience and the structure inherent in theory. This will lead to our understanding both of ourselves and of others taking on a new shape. To assimilate, for example, the meaning of the Oedipus complex, or phenomena such as repression or projective identification is—with a flash of insight into one's own experience—to come in touch with the passions and dramas that the theory seeks to provide the structure for. The force of this insight affects us so that our dispositions for continued perception and action are transformed, and, both consciously and unconsciously, we will discover that both the world and our being will unfold in new ways. On the basis of these assimilated structures it is possible once again to produce new fantasies, as happens each time the analyst intervenes or "interprets"—the difference being that now his interpretation is a fantasy founded upon his own unconscious thought processes and not on someone else's fantasy material. To assimilate the language of theory is, to me, part of the important but difficult endeavor of liberating oneself from the psychoanalyst's professional superego and, in collaboration with a more benign ego ideal, finding one's own voice as an analyst (see Grossman 1995).

And, finally, it must not be forgotten that where it truly does belong—in the separate reality of speculative and fantastic thinking—clinical theory is not annulled by the deconstructive effects of assimilation, but is retained as a territory in its own right, to be returned to from the level of evermore refined commonsense psychology that is gradually acquired.

Construction: Metapsychology

The kind of theoretical work that leads to metapsychological knowing is not unlike the work leading to clinical theory. But metapsychology has—as is indicated by its name—"raised itself" above clinical theory so that it may be viewed at a distance. One of its central functions is to keep the inclination of clinical theory to fall back into the ideological categories of commonsense psychology in check.

In order to be effective in this task, metapsychological speculation must distance itself from the language of psychology, perhaps even more so than clinical theory does. In his essay, "The Unconscious," Freud defines what he wished to see as the kernel of metapsychological knowledge: "I propose that when we have succeeded in describing a psychical process in its dynamic, topographical and economic aspects, we should speak of it as a *metapsychological* presentation" (Freud 1915:181, italics in original).

These are probably the lines most frequently quoted to present Freud's conception of metapsychology. It is certainly a precise definition, using terms exactly mirroring the content of his so-called metapsychological essays: *dynamically*, psychological phenomena are described as the result of conflict obtaining between contrary forces; *topographically*, these forces belong either to the conscious/preconscious or the unconscious system; *economically*, finally, the assumption is that these forces are determinable as to their energy content and that these energies are bound or unbound within their respective systems. Considering what is implied within such a definition, it is clear that metapsychology would not be a "second psychology." For, as is easily seen, the dynamic, topographical, and economic aspects mentioned by Freud all refer to structures and processes *totally lacking in psychological quality*. Whereas clinical theory strives to furnish a language with which we can speak of what we take to be psychic reality, metapsychology is a form of disciplined speculation concerning the fundamental structures of the mind and the nature of its processes.

To think in metapsychological terms is to think through the very foundations of psychoanalytic theory. Metapsychological reflection works like a corrective against the influence of ideology by carefully controlling the deliberations and founding hypotheses that lay the ground for clinical theory. Furthermore, through its control over clinical theory it will also define—in the double sense of "determine" and "delimit"—what in psychoanalytic experience it is possible to think about and communicate. (The reader is invited to imagine what psychoanalytic knowing would be without, for example, its fantastic metapsychological suppositions concerning repression, psychic reality, unconscious mental processes, or symptom formation.)

For psychoanalytic knowing not to end up in a vicious circle of self-confirmation, theoretical work must—at least at some decisive juncture—refrain from the temptation of basing its productions solely on the psychoanalytic experience and received psychoanalytic knowing. Here metapsychology has the obvious advantage of being able to stay open to other disciplines and enter a dialogue with, for example, linguistics, neuropsychology, or anthropology in a way that clinical theory rarely can. And, as metapsychology in fact seeks to cover a territory at the outskirts of which what one might wish to call scientific knowledge reaches its farther limits, philosophy—with its long tradition of epistemology, ontology, ethics, and value theory—is most probably the best discussion partner for psychoanalysis when involved with metapsychological construction.

The fact that it deals with the structures and workings of the mind to such a degree gives to metapsychological theory an even more obvious mythical function in comparison with clinical theory. Perhaps the clearest example of this is Freud's theory of the instincts, which has been the foremost narrative for psychoanalysis to speak of the sources of psychic activity and of psychic life. In the language of instincts the goals of the psyche have been determined, as well as its choice of objects and the conditions for its functioning. This Freud summarized as a pleasure principle.

One can only agree with Freud when he writes that "the theory of the instincts is . . . our mythology" (1933:95). This need not mean, however, that one necessarily must bow to Freud when it comes to enumerating which instincts we should assume to exist, or how we should imagine their ways of functioning. To me, the issue is wholly pragmatic: any narrative is in need of its beginning, and in theoretical work one chooses or creates the mythology that is most compatible with one's carefully elaborated convictions, and that will at the same time appear not only credible but, in the last analysis, also useful for reflecting upon clinical experience.

The possibilities of variation within the metapsychological sphere are considerable, and most important is probably not the codified theory that one ends up with, but the way one gets there. Just as the work of assimilation can be an exhaustive personal experience, the work of theoretical construction becomes deeply engaging when the theoretician must question his convictions as to what it is to be a human being, to think through such issues as the relationship between woman and man, what it means to be mad, or to scrutinize one's own sexual fantasies and practices. In all its variegated forms, theoretical work—when it is practiced with full openness to what the unconscious may surprise us with—is a thoroughgoing process that may bring about fundamental changes in the person who engages in it.

The Experiential Basis of Theoretical Work

Every so often, psychoanalysis is criticized both from within and from without for not solving its theoretical differences with reference to clinically based observational facts or data. With unrestrained contempt critics will point out how one often settles for finding "proof" for one's own standpoint by referring to what someone else has said. But, because the statements of the author referred to most probably will also lack a sound foundation in valid observations of the kind demanded, the argument is deemed equally weak.

Psychoanalysts seldom refer to observations or facts of their own or of others for the simple reason that the kind of notation asked for simply does not obtain. A scientific observation presupposes that its object, as well as its qualities and quantities, is definable in time and space. Furthermore, there is a demand that it be possible to allow more than one independent observer to arrive at the same (or at least closely similar) result in regard to the content of the observation. But what is truly decisive in the analytic situation has little to do with reproducible facts. Clinical work itself is focused upon the dialogical activity of two subjects in collaboration, and to tap such an event the analyst's watchfulness is turned inward and toward something that lets itself be known within his very being. This is a space that cannot be reached by the observing gaze, and therefore no "facts" will be produced.

Instead of referring to observations, the psychoanalyst will—just as the philosopher does—bring to mind the thinking of others, ideas resting upon the foundation of experience. For the philosopher, it is often the experience of living a life and reflecting upon its various aspects; for our part, it is the psychoanalytical experience itself. The analyst's choice of quotations is frequently dictated by his having been impressed by someone else's ability to open up the world so that it reveals itself in a new manner, or by the fact that this other person simply has made a succinct formulation he possibly wished were his own. The latter case makes it more than evident that there is a definite aesthetic moment in all theoretical work. (Beauty can definitely be the adversary of truth—such are the rules of the game. But when the two do coincide we may be faced with a statement of unusual force.)

Surely, meaningful theoretical work cannot be practiced without empirical foundations. But then, it is also important to emphasize the etymological origins of the concepts at hand. The Greek word *empereia* means *experience*, and is etymologically related to words equivalent to skillfulness, cleverness, habit, and so on. As a web of acquired dispositions, experience is the most intimate subjective knowing. From a hermeneutic perspective it would surely be an epistemological commonplace to claim that experience is a valid foundation for theoretical work that is well done. If we then remind ourselves that Plato and Aristotle used the word *teoria* in the sense of "contemplation" or "speculation," we might be able to understand theoretical work as the attentive listening to experience in combination with meditative intellectual work.

Although experience is the most intimate subjective knowing, at the same time it belongs to an unfathomable register, and it is never at hand as something ready to be discovered. Experience must be interpreted as the listening involved in theoretical work harks after the trace of something that has left our grip and has in fact been lost. Therefore, putting one's trust in myth is not the same as abandoning oneself to pure fictitiousness or unbound speculation. For good mythmaking is always in search of a formulation that can touch upon some central thematic of the analytical experience, which in itself is perhaps inaccessible. The resolve to stay faithful to the trace of the psychic reality of the analytical experience—however difficult this may be when faced with the plurality of speculative possibilities—is, to my way of thinking, the ethical precondition for good theoretical work.

So long as we are willing to assimilate theory and not just receive it, "psychoanalytic theory" can be seen as an offering of individual constructions appearing within a network of interrelated traditions. Within this network the individual psychoanalyst may seek and find something appealing, which will fit precisely his own needs—not necessarily in order to repeat the very words of received fantasy, but to find inspiration for his own continued reflection and theoretical work. With such a perspective on things, it is not really so important which theories we mingle with, and the anxiety of staying with or straying from the "correct" tradition can be seen as superfluous.

Inventing the Analysand Anew

To stay faithful to the idea of deconstruction and assimilation is to regard theory as something to be affected and stimulated by, but not to take after; it is to allow the encounter with existing theories to inspire one's own voice of commonsense psychology. A radical assimilation of theory would leave space for a moment of surprise, the importance of which in the clinical situation cannot be overestimated. The moment of surprise lies in the fact that when received knowledge has been relativized, the analyst is put in the position where he must find and invent the analysand and the analytical situation *anew every time*.

This is not a matter of in some simple sense *finding* the analysand and then telling him something, as if he were to appear spontaneously to the observing gaze. I imagine that what is taken to be "good technique" can only evolve from a blend of experience and sufficient understanding of the analysand. And with the latter I mean, above all, that we *know* him. As we saw above, getting to know someone is a result of the shared life in the matrix of communication, where I have grown acquainted with and also become part of the world of the Other. There, the language of commonsense psychology offers a form for my understanding to express itself in my capacity to say something of importance.

We can discover or find the analysand as Other only by *inventing* him—and that anew every time. Dialogical interpreting is the foremost form of this invention and its vital precondition is that *something new is created*, as, for example, when I offered my shitty brat intervention as described in the vignette above. In the same way that the work of assimilation is a central part of the process where knowledge transforms into competence, the analysand can only be discovered anew when I am creative in the very moment when I invent her. In that instant, as I abandon my own but old fantasies as well as those of others, I can meet her in a flash of momentary revelation where we both are affected.[13] That implies, for example, that one abstain from thinking in diagnostic categories. Diagnostic thinking is by nature reductionistic in that the Other is forced to conform to a mold smaller than himself.

It belongs to good analytical work that the myth or fantasy offered is allowed to grow out of the *situation itself* in a vivid way. By that I mean that the analysand's life must be understood on the basis of the inherent movement in his own narrative action, and not as a mirror image of the analyst's most cherished theories or as the result of a reductionistic hermeneutics. In dialogical interpreting the analyst acts like a subject whose actions are guided by his judgmental capacities rather than by his knowledge. The ethical gain in deconstructing any theory—even down to one's own clinical hypotheses and suppositions regarding the analysand once these have been formulated—lies in the fact that the inevitable decision is postponed to the very last moment when an intervention is called for.

Only in the unique instant of the present is it possible to discover the adequate form of expression, in an act of heedfulness where the analysand's current predicament and the analyst's spontaneous inventiveness are allowed to cooperate in the creation of a fantastic myth addressing itself to something of true import. In this way the encounter with each analysand leads to the analytical discovery—as theory *and* practice—being made anew each time. This will not come about unless a deconstructive assimilation of theory has taken place.

3

THE EPOCHS OF THE PSYCHOANALYTIC INSTITUTION

> But, strange to say, the psychoanalysts themselves
> desired respectability. They wished to set themselves
> up as part of the medical profession, and in order to
> achieve this aim they felt they had to have clinics,
> professional schools, and professional societies.
>   —S. Bernfeld 1962:466

Ever since the latter half of the nineteenth century it has been a distinctive feature of modernism that when an occupational group attained a certain size and importance and gains legitimacy by convincing the public that its methods are effective and also necessary for society, it begins to go through a process of professionalization. Thus the group starts to build member organizations, defines its specialty (together with possible subspecialties), establishes a coherent (and, in the name of scientism, preferably cumulative) knowledge base, formalizes the training curriculum, and elaborates specific criteria for graduation and certification. It introduces ethical codes and rules of conduct with the concomitant power to give warnings and reprimands and to punish by expulsion, and strives to consolidate the professional identity among the members of the corps and to gain the public's respect and confidence. Such measures are held to be the expression of the aspiration to protect the public from self-interested, ignorant, or injurious practitioners, something that in turn may be the basis for an explicit or implicit demand for monopolization of the field defined by the profession. The professionalization of the medical corps since the latter half of the nineteenth century has been so successful that it has become a model for many other professions.

From its inception, psychoanalysis evolved within a group consisting almost solely of physicians, and it was natural that one not only would try to emulate the forms for legitimization characteristic of the medical profession, but also to ally oneself directly with medicine in one's attempts to gain respectability.[1] Within the psychoanalytic movement, this process has resulted in a considerable degree of institutionalization, not in the least when it comes to such functions that concern training and certification, and it is probably not incorrect to say that "the psychoanalytical movement arranged its training system in such a way that it served the psychoanalytical institution rather than the cause. This tendency issued from the Berlin Institute" (Cremerius 1986:1074).

THE BERLIN INSTITUTE

At the Fifth International Psychoanalytic Congress in Budapest in September 1918, Sigmund Freud stated:

> It is possible to foresee that some time or another the conscience of society will awake and remind it that the poor man should have just as much right to assistance for his mind as he now has to the life-saving help offered by surgery; and that the neuroses threaten public health no less than tuberculosis, and can be left as little as the latter to the impotent care of individual members of the community. When this happens, institutions or out-patient clinics will be appointed, so that men who would otherwise give way to drink, women who have nearly succumbed under their burden of privations, children for whom there is no choice but between running wild or neurosis, may be made capable, by analysis, of resistance and of efficient work. Such treatments will be free. It may be a long time before the State comes to see these duties as urgent. Present

conditions may delay its arrival even longer. Probably these
institutions will be started by private charity. Some time or
other, however, it must come to this. [Freud 1919:167]

The same year, 1919, Max Eitingon—based upon his experience
of psychoanalytical treatment of war neuroses in a hospital setting—presented a plan for a clinic in connection with the German Psychoanalytic Society. The year after, and with the approval
of the welfare authorities (Oberndorf 1926:319), the clinic could
begin its activities, which in itself was a risky undertaking when
postwar Germany was afflicted with political strife and economic
difficulties. Thus was inaugurated the Berlin Psychoanalytic Institute, whose primary task was to offer psychoanalytic treatment
to impecunious patients. As the German Society had only a small
number of members, it became necessary to create an organization for the training of psychoanalysts to be able to provide treatment on a broader basis. In 1930, a report was published to account
for the activities of the Institute during its first ten years: *Zehn Jahre
Berliner psychoanalytisches Institut (Poliklinik und Lehranstalt)*
(Deutsche psychoanalytische Gesellschaft /DpG/ 1930). But, because this publication has never been translated into English, and
to my knowledge has been given only secondhand presentations,
more detailed knowledge of these events has been difficult to find
for anyone not prepared to turn to the German original. (Authors
of the report's different sections are: Ernst Simmel, Otto Fenichel,
Carl Müller-Braunschweig, Hans Lampl, Karen Horney, Hanns
Sachs, Franz Alexander, Sándor Radó, Siegfried Bernfeld, Felix
Boehm, J. Hárnik and Max Eitingon.) For a personal recollection
and description of the developments within the Berlin Institute,
see also Bernfeld 1962:464–467).

In the conviction that "pure" psychoanalysis—and thus no
form of therapeutic application of the analytic doctrine—was the
cure of choice to achieve permanent relief from neurotic and other
psychological difficulties, the goal was set not to compromise
when it came to methods. The impecunious were to be offered the
same treatment as could be found in the private consulting rooms,

where the patients often were of middle class and with reasonably good income.[2,3] The financing of this charity was accomplished by every member of the German Society contributing 4 percent of his or her income and agreeing to have at least one patient from the polyclinic in treatment without cost.

By the mid-twenties, the concerted voluntary input amounted to some 300 sessions per week—and by 1930 more than 400. Admirable numbers, which tell not only of the social engagement animating the second and third generations of psychoanalysts, but also of the intensive training that was carried through during these pioneering years.[4]

Between 1920 and 1930 a total of 1,995 consultations with prospective analysands had taken place. During the first years, at least, the greater part of these had been administered by Eitingon himself. On the basis of his knowledge of the volunteers, he would decide who was to take on the specific case. Even though at the start one could tell that the existing resources were insufficient to cover the needs, the realization that many of the applicants were not suited for psychoanalytic treatment came as somewhat of a surprise. However, the training of new analysts made it possible to initiate 721 analyses during the period. Of these, 241 were interrupted, and although 363 of them had led to outcomes from "improvement" to "complete recovery," 117 were still in progress at the time of publication of the Institute's report.

The patients were most often in the age range between 20 and 40 years, as were the greater number of the applicants. Twenty-nine diagnostic categories were used to classify the prospective patients; the most frequent (more than twenty cases) among those who were accepted for treatment were anxiety hysteria, character disorder, neurotic depression, hysteria, neurotic inhibition, psychopathy, schizophrenia, and obsessive neurosis. In an early account of the activities of the Institute, Max Eitingon wrote: "As time went on . . . the proletarian element diminished, while the 'intelligentsia' and the lower middle class began to preponderate" (1923:259).

The length of treatment varied between less than six months and eight years or more. On the average, though, the analyses conducted at the polyclinic must be regarded as rather short when compared with the analyses of today; most of the accomplished cases were terminated before less than twenty-four months. Still, it is possible to discern a tendency for the analyses to become lengthier toward the end of the ten-year period, a circumstance that may be explained by the fact that in 1930 as many as sixty-six analysts had graduated (this should be related to the total number of members in the International Psychoanalytic Association, which at that time was just a little over 400).

The Training System

The training program developed in Berlin during the twenties was the first organized system designed to teach future psychoanalysts. Previously, the education of a psychoanalyst had most often been rather haphazard. Not uncommonly, it would come about in such a way that a person who perhaps had read some of Freud's writings and was interested in practicing this activity called psychoanalysis would seek analytical treatment with Freud himself or someone who had been analyzed by Freud (see Falzeder 2000). Not infrequently, these analyses would last between a couple of weeks and a few months. An experience of that kind could, of course, through the selective analysis of disparate symptoms or neurotic traits, have no higher aim beyond convincing the candidate of the existence of the unconscious and at best providing him with a rudimentary measure of personal insight and a practical demonstration of the analytic technique.

Training at the Berlin Institute, which on the average took three to four years, rested upon three pillars: a personal or didactic analysis (*die Lehranalyse*); psychoanalytic work under supervision, so-called control cases (*die Kontrollanalyse*); and theoretical seminars (*der theoretische Lehrgang*). In those days—and still prevalent today—one placed the greatest emphasis upon the didactic analysis. "The didactic analysis," writes Sándor Radó in the Institute report, "serves the purpose of refining the future analyst's mental capacities as an instrument for the fulfillment of his psychological task; it shall enrich the personality by illuminating its hidden parts and strengthen its coherence" (DpG 1930:59).

Referring to Freud, Karen Horney warned against harboring too great hopes for what an analysis should be able to achieve: "Analysis . . . cannot create an ideal analyst out of just anybody, or even an averagely useful one" (DpG 1930:49). Good character and psychological talent cannot be created; such qualities can only be discovered. For that reason, the didactic analyses were regarded as "trial analyses," and not before the didactic analysis was terminated could it be decided whether the applicant was fit to go on and become a training candidate in a more strict sense, which is to say attend the theoretical seminars and start conducting control analyses. In this way, the function of the applicant's analyst—the so-called didactic or training analyst—became of central importance in that it was on the basis of his report to the training committee that the applicant would be accepted for or barred from further training. The earliest didactic analyses can be said to have been of a "friendly" character, but they now became a formal institution within the psychoanalytic movement, and in addition—as we shall see in the following chapter—a fateful factor in its future development.

The training candidates could partake in the Institute's program with two different aims. To the first group belonged those who sought a professional career as psychoanalysts in private practice. To the second belonged those who were to utilize their psychoanalytic knowledge within their original occupations. These could be physicians, social workers, teachers, lawyers, or ministers. A number of special seminars were arranged for this group. It was thought that for those who aimed at becoming psychoanalysts medical schooling and experience were the best preconditions for training, while at the same time some held the view that there were persons with differing backgrounds who could have knowledge, experience, and personal qualities making them suited for the profession. One extra requirement demanded of those lacking medical training was that they should have had some clinical experience working with mental patients.

In addition to the "true" training candidates, the Institute would also enlist a group of people called "listeners" or "students" (*Hörer*). These persons would not conduct control cases, nor would they attend the clinically oriented technical seminars. But apart from that, they had access to all the courses offered. They came from a variety of professions, and the purpose of letting them attend was to spread psychoanalytic knowledge to new fields— to make of psychoanalysis a cultural factor, as it were. In the same vein, a large number of lectures were given to the general public on the clinical aspects of psychoanalysis and its application within other disciplines.

As was mentioned, the candidates could embark upon theoretical studies only after they had undergone a didactic analysis. The theoretical training was aimed at providing basic command of the psychoanalytical body of knowledge. Due to a lack of experienced teachers, it took several years before a well-designed curriculum was worked out. There was a widespread skepticism among the teachers as to whether psychoanalytic knowledge as yet was empirically well founded and tested enough and its concepts so well developed that they were fit to be transmitted in a more systematic way. To a degree, this standpoint seems to have been based upon the view that psychoanalysis did indeed propagate something that was totally new and therefore was unable to borrow from other disciplines or find its roots within any existing tradition. Instead, teachers wished to await the natural and necessarily protracted development of the concepts taking place as the empirical foundations for psychoanalysis gradually grew stronger.

Thus, the theoretical lectures given at the Institute were at first only loosely connected to the demands of the training itself. Apart from a common ground consisting of the theory of sexuality, the theory of dreams, and neuroses, a variegated list of lectures was offered that seems to have been dictated by the current interests of the teachers involved—one simply used what was presently at hand. Gradually, this was to change.

During the very first years, the organization of the Institute's lecturing activities had been under the direction of Karl Abraham, Max Eitingon, and Ernst Simmel. In 1923 a training committee within the German Psychoanalytic Society was founded under the auspices of Eitingon, with the task of handling all possible training issues. One of the committee's first missions was to establish guidelines for the training program. Subsequent to that, the day-to-day work of the committee consisted of: (1) selecting candidates for training; (2) evaluating the didactic analyses (based upon the reports from the training analysts) and deciding whether the applicant will be allowed to continue his training; (3) setting the curriculum of seminars and appointing the proper teachers; and (4) contributing (after 1925) to the tasks of the International Training Commission of the IPA.

At the inception of the autumn semester in 1927, a compulsory curriculum was introduced, where, above all, the theoretical lectures and seminars were harmonized within a systematic order of training. With that, a gradual shift took place within the theoretical training from lectures to more practically oriented seminars. The complete curriculum now entailed the still-well-known moments of didactic analysis, theoretical studies (two years), and the so-called control cases, which were to be conducted under supervision together with a "technical colloquium."

The aim of the control cases was to deepen the knowledge of the practical handling of psychoanalytical treatment acquired by the candidate when he had undergone his didactic analysis. It had been observed that certain complications would be bound to arise when the analyst-to-be was to assume a new role—from the analysand's "passive" position to the active one of the analyst.[5] The specific conditions of the psychoanalytic treatment did, however, forbid any immediate "help" or "aid" to the practitioner. For example, the candidate could not perform his work before a colleague whose task was to offer his best advice in the very moment of discovery. Instead, the "control case" was established, a system in which the candidate privately meets his patient and then regularly presents his work to an experienced analyst for guidance. The guide was at this time designated as *Kontrollana-lytiker*—today we say "supervisor."

The control analyses were soon to be extended into technical colloquiums or seminars. In these groups—supervised by one of the appointed teachers of the Institute—the candidates could give detailed presentations of their own cases and, in shared discussions, develop their understanding of their own work while at the same time gaining further knowledge through the work of others. Not least important was, of course, the experience supplied by the teacher in the group. As the training program developed, the technical seminar grew to the point where it was necessary to partition it into smaller groups.

To make it possible for applicants lacking the financial background to undergo their didactic analysis, a grant was instituted in 1924 by taxing the members of the Berlin Society, in addition to private donations. The candidate would then contract to later repay the amount borrowed. By 1930, nine such analyses had been carried to their completion. With the help of donations, a psychoanalytical library encompassing some 400 volumes had also been founded, together with a reference library belonging to the Institute and carrying 1,200 volumes.

With the advent of Hitler's *Machtübernahme* in 1933, the activities of the Berlin Institute were gradually to diminish, while at the same time the number of applicants to the polyclinic lessened only marginally. During the years 1932 to 1934 Bernfeld, Eitingon, Fenichel, Harnik, Reik, and Simmel had left Germany (Müeller-Braunschweig 1935:248). With the hope of saving the presence of psychoanalysis in Nazi Germany, and at the recommendation of Ernest Jones, the German Psychoanalytical Society (DgP) had agreed to expel all of its Jewish members. In 1936 the *Deutsche Institut für psychologische Forschung* was founded by Matthias Heinrich Göring (cousin of Hermann), and later that same year the DgP was incorporated into the "Göring Institute." At the same time the "Jewish" term "psychoanalysis" was now replaced with the more "Aryan" "deep psychotherapy," and Jews were forbidden to either practice psychotherapy or undergo such treatment (Roudinesco and Plon 1997:385; 711).[6]

International Developments

The overarching structure of the Berlin Institute has been the model for practically all subsequent psychoanalytic training. In most psychoanalytic societies the world over (IPA and IFPS), the compulsory curriculum will encompass (at least) these three elements: (1) the personal analysis; (2) theoretical seminars; and (3) supervised cases.[7] The first of these regular institutes was established in 1924 in Vienna, based on what had been learned in Berlin. Thus, one did not only set up a training facility, but also a polyclinic (Deutsch 1932:256; the idea of giving technical colloquiums seems to have originated in Vienna /Szasz 1958/).[8]

The first step toward a general internationalization of psychoanalytic training was taken at the IPA's ninth congress in 1925 at Bad Homburg, where it was decided that every component society of the IPA should appoint a special committee responsible for training activities. Individual members were henceforth advised against training new analysts on their own (see Eitingon 1925:131). In connection with that, an "International Training Commission" (ITC) was also formed. In the IPA statutes of 1928 the above decree was augmented to the effect that the ITC should be "the central agent of the I.P.A. on all matters connected with instruction in psycho-analysis" (*International Journal of Psycho-Analysis* 9:158). That same year it was decreed that the component societies should establish a general set of rules by which to manage their respective training systems.

After that, rapid centralization and bureaucratization set in. Via the ITC, the IPA gained almost total control of all training activities. In illustration of this, in the so-called "Standing Rules of the ITC in Relation to Training Institutes and Training Centres" issued in 1934, it is stated that "The regulations, or changes in the regulations, of any Training Institute shall be submitted to the I.T.C. for approval" (*International Journal of Psycho-Analysis* 16:246).[9] For known historical reasons, Americans do not easily take instructions from Europe, and in the long run they could not accept what they perceived as overpowering ukases from the IPA and the ITC.[10]

The decisive power struggle was to a great extent played out around those analysts who did not have medical training. The disputes took on a formal character when Theodore Reik, a prominent member of the Vienna Society and a layman, was prosecuted for quackery due to a maltreatment complaint filed by a former analysand. Reik was acquitted—mostly because the complainant was deemed to be unreliable—but while the case was in the courts Freud had written a book in defense of nonphysicians: *The Question of Lay Analysis* (Freud 1926).

Freud's book made a latent conflict rise to the surface.[11] While Freud insistently maintained that psychoanalysis indeed needed knowledgeable and gifted persons from other disciplines, there were strong forces who regarded psychoanalysis as a branch of medicine, and in line with that held the view that only physicians should be admitted to the training institutes. In 1927, the issue was widely discussed and was specifically addressed at the tenth IPA congress in Innsbruck the same year. After continued discussions a compromise was reached, and it was established that each component society would have the right to decide upon the rules for admission to its training program.[12]

This, however, gave rise to the difficulty that the status of graduated psychoanalyst was not automatically recognized when a lay analyst moved to a country whose society only accepted physicians. This was solved by making it possible for individual analysts to become direct members of the IPA—and not via a component society. The American Psychoanalytic Association (APA) protested vehemently against this on the grounds that they felt it to be an incursion upon their independence. At the IPA's fifteenth congress in Paris in 1938, the APA threatened to leave the IPA unless: (1) the ITC was dismantled; (2) the direct member-ship of analysts moving to the United States was withdrawn; (3) the IPA was to handle only scientific issues; and (4) that it was to relinquish all administrative power (Jones 1957:322).[13]

In practice, the conflict was solved through the intervention of the Second World War. After the war a great part of European psychoanalysis had been crushed and the Americans no longer felt any threat coming from the European authority. They were now free to do as they wished and therefore could afford to main-tain friendly relations with the IPA, which had its headquarters in England, where European psychoanalysis, despite the war, had had the greatest possibilities of surviving and developing. As to the International Commission, a few years after the end of the war Balint summarized the whole issue with the words: "One does not know whether the I.T.C. still exists in reality, or on paper only, or even not at all" (1948:168). At the sixteenth psychoanalytic congress in Zürich in 1949, the existing state of affairs was con-firmed as the new bylaws of the IPA tacitly accepted the Ameri-can resolution of 1938 (Knight 1953:201). But, ironically, the APA's victorious struggle against the oppressive European authority was to result in a considerably stricter regime than what psychoanaly-sis in Europe had ever witnessed.

THE THREE EPOCHS OF THE PSYCHOANALYTIC INSTITUTION

In an article from 1948, "On the Psychoanalytic Training Sys-tem," Michael Balint points out that until then—which is to say more than twenty-five years after the Berlin Institute had begun its activities—practically nothing had been published that seri-ously discussed the various problems connected with psychoana-lytic training. Balint attributes this long silence in part to the risk that if the training were to be seriously scrutinized it would be-come clear that certain training analysts had not had an adequate training analysis themselves, and in part to the fact that one would have to evaluate the efficacy of training analyses on the whole. The latter issue could possibly lead to some grave questioning of all psychoanalytic training.

I will save Balint's comments on these topics for later, and in this chapter instead emphasize the periodization of the psychoanalytic training system that he suggested and that has been referred to by many after him. I will refrain from using his denominations, and instead refer to the suggested time periods as the first, the second, and the third "epoch" of the psychoanalytic institution. With small modifications, these epochs could very well also cover what might be meant by the epochs or eras of the psychoanalytic movement on the whole, but I am not going to go deeper into that.

> From the year 1902 onwards, a number of young doctors gathered round me with the express intention of learning, practising and spreading the knowledge of psycho-analysis. The stimulus came from a colleague who had himself experienced the beneficial effects of analytic therapy. Regular meetings took place on certain evenings at my house, discussions were held according to certain rules and the participants endeavoured to find their bearings in this new and strange field of research and to interest others in it. [Freud 1914b:25]

The first epoch of the psychoanalytic institution began during the first years of the twentieth century when Freud gathered a group of disciples in a setting without any demands for formal training—an issue that seems to have been of little interest to Freud. Those who wished to approach psychoanalysis were in most cases accepted without rigorous inspection, and most personal analyses were—as was mentioned above—brief and not very deep. There was no curriculum for theoretical studies, and any new member was expected to read on his own, and above all partake in some form of collegial gathering or seminar where scientific discussions would have some of the function that the supervisory institution later would carry.

Szasz emphasizes that the first epoch mainly coincides with a time when psychoanalysis had not yet won acceptance by the general public (Szasz 1958:599),[14] which means that those who gathered came neither for fame nor for money, something that would become much more prevalent during the second and perhaps even more so during the third epoch. The pioneers of the first epoch were spirited with the pure joy of discovery and were more engaged in *seeking* the truth than transforming it into a system of knowledge: in other words, professionalization had not yet begun. As we saw above, the Berlin Institute was faced with just such a decision: Was it at all possible to regard the body of psychoanalytic knowledge as a coherent system to be transmitted through institutions of tutelage?

The second epoch started with the founding of the Berlin Institute in 1920. Balint laconically states that while there had been great hopes of providing psychoanalytic treatment to the broad masses, the only thing that had been successful was the establishment of a system of training. Therapy for the many and the poor was to vanish totally. The same happened with another one of the Institute's ambitions: research. Results in that respect, wrote Balint (1948:168), were so poor that they scarcely deserve mention.

The only really strong and lively tendency during the second epoch was a striving for control and centralization. Balint regretted the great mistakes made by the ITC, which, with European haughtiness, had sought to subdue the APA into a condition of dependency, while at the same time he deplored the latter's "unnecessarily fierce rebellion" together with the "American Declaration of Independence," which was to become the start of the third epoch of the psychoanalytical institution. The inner effects of these forces of power were that the psychoanalyst would now obey a paternalistic authority, something that necessarily would already be inculcated in the training candidate through active persuasion, with the aim of making him accept anything that his superiors taught him and that he would in the end identify with the authority itself.

The third epoch—which in Balint's historiography commences with the outbreak of World War II—is the very time of harvest for these tendencies. No longer does anyone even try to pretend that psychoanalytic training should serve the superordinate aim of providing the masses with polyclinical treatment. The training institution—and its overarching aim to ensure the continuation and continued expansion of the profession—has become its own foundation of legitimization and the hub around which most of the activities of psychoanalytic societies revolve.

According to the analysis offered by Balint, it was perhaps predominantly the dramatic breaks between Freud and Adler and Jung during the second decade of the twentieth century that laid the ground for the fatal centralization of power that was to follow. Animated with the expansive spirit prevailing during the first epoch, many of Freud's disciples wished to develop ideas of their own.[15] Balint quotes Freud in a rather early text as he addresses the very danger brought about by this tendency toward independence: "Yet I felt that there must be someone at the head. I knew only too well the pitfalls that lay in wait for anyone who became engaged in analysis, and hoped that many of them might be avoided if an authority could be set up who would be prepared to instruct and admonish" (Freud 1914b:43).

Balint takes notice especially of Freud's use of the word "admonish" (*Abmahnung*) and interprets it to mean that if psychoanalysis really wants to avoid future divisions, coming generations must at least to a degree refrain from defending their own positions and instead submit to authority and exercise self-discipline. The psychoanalytic movement would form and develop through its future analysts identifying with its forebears and their ideas.[16]

With the third generation of psychoanalysts (Freud being the first and his earliest followers the second generation), starting to appear by the mid-1920s in Berlin and the United States, this authority began to wither. For those who did not break with Freud, his presence still constituted a unifying force for the psychoanalytic movement—and this to an extent that in our day may be difficult to appreciate. Therefore, the third epoch of the psychoanalytic institution is not initiated until his death in 1939 and with the general loss of authority that fell upon the movement as a whole. Pent-up forces could now be set free, and during and after the Second World War more and more deep-seated ideological and theoretical differences of opinion resulted in the movement splitting up into a number of competing schools. The most powerful of these was ego psychology, which was to dominate not only the American psychoanalytic societies, but also psychoanalysis in Germany, which had been robbed of its identity after its fatal collaboration with the Nazis.

During the war, a distressing battle had taken place in England between the followers of Anna Freud and those of Melanie Klein. Anna Freud's version of the analytic doctrine retained common points with American ego psychology, whereas the Kleinian movement remained a closed group for a long period, with followers mostly in South America and Spain. Between these two poles dividing English psychoanalysis, a third force was formed by the mid-forties, the so-called Middle Group, which chose not to side with either of the two contestants. Apart from its national political function, internationally the Middle Group has mostly been identified as the spokesman for so-called object relations theory.

Through the presence of the faithful Freud disciple, Marie Bonaparte, a generally ego psychological orientation was maintained in the Paris Society. In 1953, however, a break took place when a number of central figures left the Society; perhaps the most well known of these were Daniel Lagache and Jacques Lacan. The seceders had not taken into account the fact that they would lose their membership in the IPA when they left the Society, and only after ten years of tough negotiations with the IPA were some of the defectors, together with their followers, allowed renewed membership through the founding of the French Psychoanalytical Society. For that reason there have been two IPA groups in Paris since 1964.

Because of his unorthodox and "wild" way of handling the length of sessions, and his unconditional demand of retaining his status as training analyst and teacher in the new French Society, Lacan was excluded from it. Together with his most devout followers he instead founded the *École freudienne* in 1965, a "school" that lacked many of the characteristics typical of the IPA societies: no fixed curriculum, no training analyst institution, and, not least important, the ideological conviction that a psychoanalyst can only authorize himself. With the widely known seminars that Lacan had held ever since the break in 1953 as its intellectual pivot and primary object of transference, the *École freudienne* developed during the seventies into what might be likened to a national movement, with considerable coverage in the media and a great impact on cultural life in France. Today, the Lacanian doctrine— if it is at all possible to speak of something like that—exercises an influence on the dominant IPA ideology that thus far remains difficult to assess.[17]

When it comes to training issues it is interesting to note—just as did Balint—how, for example, the dramatic conflict over clinical theory between the Anna Freudians and the Kleinians in England in no way evidenced any differences in training cultures. On the whole, during the third epoch practically all psychoanalytic training has become more uniform, characterized by similar requirements and institutional forms, as if the analytic movement, regardless of theoretical conviction, had been blinded by its institutional demands for authority and power over its members. This in itself has not gone unnoticed, but as is so often the case, institutions have an uncanny capacity to withstand criticism, leaving a clear power structure to prevail and crystallize into the kind of dogmatism already discussed by Balint in 1948.

> It is not enough to insist that every analyst must have a personal analysis. The law-makers will be strongly tempted—and pressured—to qualify and define the meaning of the term "personal analysis." Next they will figure out how long the analysis must take, how many weekly sessions it must have, which analysts are qualified to give it and which are not, and on and on in this strain. Soon we find ourselves in our present situation, with the certain promise of worse to come if this law-making trend is not curbed.
>
> In 1924, when I saw the legislators so passionately at work in Berlin, I thought they were, perhaps naturally, animated by the spirit of the Prussian army. Since those days I have come

to understand that institutionalization has nothing to do with that specific spirit, but that the laying down of laws is a hobby of psychoanalysts everywhere. [Bernfeld 1962:478–479]

PSYCHOANALYSIS AND PSYCHIATRY

Jones relates how, at the end of the thirties a rumor was circulating in the United States to the effect that Freud had changed his mind concerning lay analysts and now advocated that only medical men should have access to the analytical profession. In a letter of July 5, 1938, Freud answers a direct question on this topic thus: "The fact is, I have never repudiated [my earlier] views and I insist on them even more intensely than before, in the face of the obvious American tendency to turn psycho-analysis into a mere house-maid of psychiatry" (quoted in Jones 1957:323).

Peace among nations also meant peace among psychoanalysts, and this would turn out to have fateful consequences that are foreboded in Freud's letter. During the decades following the end of World War II, American ego psychology was to reach a dominating position within the international psychoanalytic movement, not in the least due to the large number of American analysts and their prolific theoretical production.[18] Through this American dominance the medical paradigm was to be maintained and spread as the metaphysical and social foundation for psychoanalysis, a circumstance that justifies a short historical digression to trace the outlines of the medical influence upon American psychoanalysis after the Second World War.[19]

This is no local American issue, and it is not at all unreasonable to speculate that the dissemination of psychoanalysis would never have been so extensive and its survival so enduring had it not entered some kind of alliance with medicine. For only medicine has enjoyed the authority that can bestow legitimacy and respectability on the analytic project.[20] Even though the basic fit between these two ways of thinking has been rather poor, the relative freedom allotted to psychoanalysis has been great enough for it to develop decently under the aegis of medicine, although perhaps in certain respects its development has been somewhat stunted.

It is probably the very fact that psychoanalysis was connected to the pragmatism of medicine that has contributed most to allowing it to gain the public's confidence, for with such an ally it was perceived to be in possession of scientifically founded knowledge. To this must be added the role allotted to psychoanalysis in general consciousness, in part due to the fact that in certain influential social strata a relatively large number of people were in analytic treatment and could give evidence of their experience, and in part as a cultural impact in society at large through its presence in books, films, and cartoons, together with the assimilation of analytic knowing by the man in the street.[21]

What is respected in the United States tends to deposit as authority in Europe, and on both sides of the Atlantic the consolidation of the psychoanalytic process of professionalization, which had begun with the establishment of the Berlin Institute during the twenties gradually took place. And although it is true that European psychoanalysis has never had such close ties to psychiatry as in America, a significant number of European analysts have been psychiatrists. I would therefore like to suggest that practically everywhere the psychoanalytic process of professionalization has been filtered through some form of cohabitation with psychiatry.

The first clear signs of a rapprochement between American psychoanalysis and psychiatry had already appeared in the twenties when the APA and the American Psychiatric Association began to hold their spring congresses in the same city, temporally coordinated and with certain joint arrangements.[22] What was limited during the thirties and also in the resolution of 1938 to the explicit ambition to limit the accreditation of psychoanalysts to physicians was now codified in the APA bylaws that were approved in 1946 and where it was decreed that all new members— even those who had been trained in Europe and moved to the United States—must be medical doctors. In an address given in

1942 by Karl Menninger, chairman of the APA, it is abundantly clear what the relationship between psychoanalysis and psychiatry looked like at this time: after having established that the American Psychiatric Association is scientifically the parent organization of the APA, he goes on to say that "we are physicians first, psychiatrists second, and psychoanalysts third" (1942:290).[23]

In 1952 the societies within the APA comprised 485 members in all, and out of these not more than about 30 were laymen (simultaneously there were about 900 candidates in training). At the same time 82 percent of these 485 members were also members of the American Psychiatric Association. For the sake of comparison it may be mentioned that a few years later, in 1960, there were 604 analysts in Europe, and out of these, 370 were physicians/psychiatrists and 234 were laymen; simultaneously 506 candidates were in training (van der Leeuw 1962:277).

During the Second World War a large number of the body of psychoanalysts had served in wartime psychiatry and had there given proof of a level of competence and dexterity that seemed almost unattainable to the younger psychiatrists. As a result of these strong impressions the immediate postwar period saw a veritable rush of psychiatrists to the analytical institutes. Bird (1968:520) speculates that what actually interested these applicants was not so much becoming psychoanalysts, but rather to be what he calls "super psychiatrists" of the kind they had encountered in war psychiatry. From these recruits arose a large corps of psychiatrists/analysts who were to become both influential within American psychoanalysis and the leading group behind the dynamic psychiatry that evolved after the war (see below).[24,25]

In the fifties, American psychiatrists were divided between those who were biologically oriented and those who were psychologically and socially oriented. The former relied mainly upon such measures as electroshock therapy, medication with the newly discovered psychopharmacological substances, and neurosurgical interventions. To the latter group, training to become a psychoanalyst was a must and a sign of acceptance and success. Within this group there was what Szasz has called a "caste-system," the highest caste being composed of full-fledged analysts. Among these, in turn, there was a subgroup of even higher standing: the training analysts. On a lower rung of the ladder stood those who had not had analytical training proper, but who wanted to count as belonging to the "analytically oriented" or "dynamic" psychiatrists. (That someone landed in this group could be due to the fact that she or he had not qualified for selection to analytic training or was unfortunate enough to live too far away from an analytic institute.)

The connection with psychiatry gave rise to a new kind of psychoanalyst: the part-time practitioner who conducts psychoanalysis part of the day and during the remaining hours does something else, like working at a hospital, teaching, or administrating. Before the war the part-time practitioner had been an almost unknown phenomenon, while at the same time the mutual dependency between psychoanalysts and psychiatry had developed to the point where one good reason for seeking analytic training was that it would make it easier later to reach the position of teacher in psychiatry! As has been noted by Bird (1968), a considerable number of those who applied for psychoanalytic training after the war did not do this for the sake of becoming practicing analysts, but were instead intent on doing work that was far removed from the clinical realities of psychoanalysis.

Dorn refers to an unpublished work by T. Webster: "Career Decisions and Professional Self-image of Medical Students" from 1966, where it is clear that males who chose medical training in the United States during the sixties belonged to the most high-achieving tenth of all college students. Of those students who did *not* choose medicine, more than four times that many (46 percent) stressed the importance of "original and creative" work opportunities than did those who chose medicine. "As psychoanalysts we should concern ourselves with the possible significance to our field that this siphoning-away of creative individuals represents. Does medicine tend to attract the intellectually endowed who shy away from creativity (possibly avoiding contact with the unconscious)?" (Dorn 1969:245).

One further important consequence of the cohabitation between analysis and psychiatry has been a gradual shift in the
understanding of "analyzability," and with it a noticeable theoretical and clinical trend. Before the Second World War the average psychoanalyst—like Freud himself—had little contact with
clinical psychiatry. To the extent that she or he would accept
patients belonging to any other diagnostic groups than the classic neuroses (even these would practically always be treated with
the standard psychoanalytic method), those who did not pass that
test were regarded as unanalyzable and were most often referred
to psychiatric treatment. The exposure to psychiatric realities after
the war would, of necessity, lead to different attempts at modify-
ing the analytical method and developing its theories so that it
would be possible to treat patients belonging to a wider scope of
diagnostic categories.[26]

The dynamic psychiatry—endowed with an unmistakable
welfare ideology—that would evolve from these premises was
guided by great optimism, inventiveness, and a strong wish to
help. It started out during the forties and culminated some time
during the seventies.[27] Theoretically, during the fifties, this development at first contributed to the expansion of ego psychology, but the protracted exposure to such diagnostic categories as
borderline conditions, narcissistic personality disorders, and psy-
choses would eventually demand a theory that would reach deeper
and touch upon earlier stages of personality development. Thus
came about a kind of crisis for ego psychology, while at the same
time some camps directed their gaze toward the so-called object
relations theories of Melanie Klein and the British School.

Typical of the psychiatric welfare ideology was a pragmatic
stance which, when it came to psychoanalysis, always threatened
to yield negative consequences. Whereas dynamic psychiatry has
deepened and widened its methods, the distinction between psychotherapy and psychoanalysis has tended to become blurred: the
more or less presuppositionless investigation of the meaningful
connections within a mind has threatened to be surpassed by more
symptom-oriented methods guided by explicit health goals (see

Dorn 1969:246; Gitelson 1963:525; Knight 1953:216).[28] The effects on psychoanalysis proper are apparent as both candidates and graduated analysts must adapt to psychiatric demands, and psychoanalytic institutions no longer remain the propagators of an exclusive and esoteric activity such as "pure" psychoanalysis.[29]

The Demise of the APA as a Medical Bastion

As a result of the APA's exclusion of dissidents from its own ranks and of protestations against its absolutism, a number of psychoanalytic societies independent of the APA/IPA were formed in the United States during the forties and the fifties. Some of these were to distance themselves vehemently from the prevailing ego psychological and medical dominance within American psychoanalysis, while still others were just as "mainstream," but with considerably greater leeway for who could become a psychoanalyst and how one is allowed to think. Within the IPA there had always been analysts who did not identify with the strict rules of admission and who therefore would provide training analyses and supervision for these groups, whereby it would often be possible to maintain a standard equal to that of the APA and IPA societies.

At the beginning of the sixties, some of the independent societies acted to form a separate international: the International Federation of Psychoanalytic Societies (IFPS).[30] Within the component societies of the IFPS—situated in the United States, Europe, and South America—the original opposition against the APA's medical autocracy has found expression in how training systems have remained open to psychologists as well. But, as is often the case with defectors from an organization as "catholic" as the IPA, the IFPS has generally been regarded as a weaker authority with a lesser degree of legitimacy. In part, this is probably because the IFPS maintained lower requirements for matriculation for a protracted period. During the eighties, however, the IFPS made a general revision of its statutes and approved minimal standards that on the whole equaled those of the IPA. As a consequence of that, it seems, analysts belonging to the IFPS started to figure among the references of IPA publications.

To psychologists who wished to train at any of the APA societies the doors had been completely shut—the exception being a small number who had been admitted with the express aim of becoming psychoanalytical researchers (and *not* clinicians!). This state of affairs changed rapidly during the eighties, when a psychoanalytical section was established within the American Psychological Association. Later, four members of the section filed a complaint against the APA, the IPA, and two component societies of the APA for defying the American antitrust legislation and obstructing free competition between physicians and psychologists by refusing the latter access to their training. In 1985—only nine months after the complaint had been filed—the IPA reacted by changing its statutes so that psychoanalytical groups and societies could apply for direct membership without recourse to the APA.

After a couple of years of tough negotiations—when the IPA lawyers actually threatened to disclose information from the defendants' own analyses with training analysts belonging to the IPA to prove their unanalyzability (sic; see Schneider and Desmond 1994:325), an agreement was finally reached in 1989, the most important element of which was that psychologists and other suitable nonmedical clinical practitioners were now admissible to the APA's training systems and thereafter could apply for membership. In conjunction with that, three American societies that had chosen not to join the IFPS were connected at the IPA congress in Rome. In 1993 these groups in turn established an American organization of their own: IPS, Coalition of Independent Psychoanalytic Societies in the United States (Freedman and Sanville 1999).

But all was not smooth sailing because both the APA and the IPA embarked upon a crude tactic of postponement aimed against other groups and individuals who sought membership and/or training, while setting up new demands going far beyond what had originally been stated in the agreement, forcing the psychologists to threaten with renewed legal action (Karon 1994). That the APA would not welcome the new conditions unanimously was to be expected. The lack of gentlemanly behavior on the part of the IPA, however, is considerably more surprising and must be ascribed to some very mixed feelings among its leading figures as to how the presence of the new groups would affect the central organization. Today the parties seem to have reached an equilibrium, and perhaps Karon is correct in writing that "the lawsuit is probably the best thing that has happened to the [APA] and the IPA in many years, because it has brought an influx of bright energetic young psychologists into those organizations, and into what had been the mainstream of psychoanalysis" (352).[31]

4

Central Functions in Psychoanalytic Training

> It almost looks as if analysis were the third of those
> "impossible" professions in which one can be sure
> beforehand of achieving unsatisfying results. The other
> two, which have been known much longer, are educa-
> tion and government.
>
> —S. Freud 1937:248

Freud wrote this at the end of the thirties, burdened as he was at the time by a certain pessimism as to the psychoanalytical project, which seems to have been with him for some while. If it is true that psychoanalysis and education both are "impossible," it must be especially difficult to handle the combination of educating psychoanalysts, with its implied exercise of power, and maintaining the very values that such training is designed to promulgate. That complication is like a shadow that psychoanalysis casts over its own activity—and this is the topic of this and the following chapter.

Generally speaking, psychoanalytic training is much the same in all countries, and rests upon the tripartite model we can recognize from the Berlin Institute: (1) a personal psychoanalysis; (2) theoretical seminars; (3) psychoanalytic work under supervision from a training analyst. In some societies certain matriculation requirements are added, like writing and/or reading a paper. A complete training from admission to graduated psychoanalyst will typically take some five to ten years.

Psychoanalytic training—which almost without exception takes place within private institutes and without economic funding from the community—is undertaken with great sacrifice on the part of the candidate. For that reason the candidate must conduct his studies along with some other "regular" work, and it is practically inevitable that the total number of hours will exceed what is regarded to be a normal week of work. In addition to that, it has been reported that the greater portion of the candidate's total training expenses (quite apart from the loss of income due to the hours spent on studies) is spent on the compulsory training analysis. In a survey conducted in 1971 it was established that at some institutes the candidates would spend up to 50 percent of their available time and money on their training (Terman 1972:48).

> A vocation may be strong, but the trainings are tougher than they were, and the logistical problems have a dreadful reality. Students often look, and are, completely exhausted as the breaks between training terms approach. Some marriages do not survive personal psychotherapy or analysis, and some of the students' children become disturbed. [Coltart 1993:6–7; see also A. Freud 1971:230]

Candidates are often recruited at the age of forty or older, and Wallerstein states that at some institutes it is not uncommon that individuals will graduate only after they are fifty (1978:499). Faure-Pragier, at the Paris Psychoanalytical Society, reports candidates who are as old as sixty! (1999:76).[1] The generally advanced age of candidates leads to the newly graduated having relatively little time left for learning the praxis of analysis to such an extent that they will be able to find their own voice and make a contribution to analytical thinking.

In what follows I shall map some of the central functions of psychoanalytic training (without regard for their being conscious or unconscious, explicit or tacit), the effects of which—in particular in how this manifests itself in the form of the psychoanalytical superego complex—we will investigate in Chapter 5. These functions are sought within the following moments of analytic training: the selection of candidates, the training analysis, the supervised cases, and the theoretical seminars.

THE SELECTION OF CANDIDATES

We lack the criteria for prediction, we do not know exactly what the qualities are which go into the making of a good analyst, what accomplishments are required for our daily work.

—P. J. Van Der Leeuw 1968:164

In selecting for psychoanalytic training, we are doing something we do not (precisely) know in order to achieve something we cannot (precisely) describe.

—W. Kappelle 1996:1229

Which groups are interested in us and which ones do we wish to deal with? Who are the most suited to profit by the training? Which qualities do we find indispensable for a "good enough" analyst? Who are the best suited for doing analytical work? What possibilities have we for making reliable predictions concerning those who apply? Questions like these guide candidate selection and admission procedures.

During the first epoch of psychoanalysis questions like these were, as we have seen, rarely posed—at least not in such a clear way. Future analysts would appoint themselves by joining the movement, seeking a personal analysis, and starting to take patients in treatment. They had an abundance of that quality that Anna Freud (1983:260–261) by the end of her life (i.e., during the third epoch) felt that one tended to pay least attention to when selecting candidates: curiosity and an ardent interest in how people function, both when in harmony with themselves and when suffering from inner dissonance.

During the second epoch of the analytical institution, when the process of professionalization had just barely begun, Horney wrote, as we have seen, in the report of the Berlin Institute, that a didactic analysis "cannot create an ideal analyst out of just anybody" (DpG 1930:49). Not everyone is suited to become a psychoanalyst—in all probability not even if one harbors the ardent interest referred to by Anna Freud. Institutes were on the lookout for those who were especially suited, but did not know how to discern which ones they were without subjecting promising applicants to "trial analyses" (*Probeanalyse*). Only when the trial analysis was terminated was it possible to decide whether the applicant was indeed suited for admission.

This was evidently not a very economical procedure, as a considerable number of training analysts would be tied up with analyses that in many cases would not lead to the desired result: a future colleague. In addition, it must have seemed ethically suspect to encourage the commencement of analytical treatments whose aim was to separate the suitable from the nonsuitable. I have not been able to find these two considerations in the literature, but I assume that they must have occurred. It is, for example, quite possible to interpret an observation by Greenacre as a weak reflection of the economic argument: she writes in passing that after the Second World War there were not enough training analysts in the United States to receive all applicants (1961:39). The economic factor must have necessitated the demand that one must *know* something concerning the suitability of applicants *before* embarking upon a training analysis.

Since the forties, an abundant literature has appeared dealing with the selection of candidates.[2] It is somewhat disconcerting to see how the same basic questions and issues are repeated and varied without much new being said and without the fundamental problems being solved. I mention this only to point out how in all probability the selection of candidates is the most difficult part of the training system to organize. And that is something no one seems to agree on, while at the same time, seemingly no one ever gives up attempts at bettering the system or at least entertaining the hope of one day having better methods: "Devising requirements and judging qualifications exert an uncanny attraction upon members of the psychoanalytic educational community. It is no exaggeration to say that more time has been spent on these subjects by educational committees and by the Board of Professional Standards than on any other subject" (Arlow 1982:6).

The most obvious signs of this ambition are the repeated attempts at constructing lists—the "catalogues of virtue"—to cover all the desirable qualities an analyst should have and the norms of excellence he must live up to. Certain virtues are always recurrent, as for example the capacity for empathy, the capacity for identification, the interest in and strength to encounter the effects of one's unconscious, self-knowledge, and so on. Other virtues— which are equally important or pertinent—appear more seldom: the capacity for attention, the capacity for letting oneself be taken by surprise, a sense of responsibility, the capacity to capture the point of urgency in every moment (Strachey 1934:150). To the list of more rarely mentioned virtues, I could add the capacity for selecting the patients one is really suited for and the capacity for theoretical work (in the sense developed in Chapter 2).

Some commentators will make heavier demands. Thus, for example, Greenson writes that the sought-for qualities presuppose "persons of unusual sensitivity, personality, and character" (1966:14). Lampl-De Groot holds that "integrity of character" is indispensable (1954:184), a point that Heimann laconically comments on by saying that integrity of character is a particularly rare quality. She adds that if we demand such qualities of those seeking analytic training this will inevitably strengthen the general view that psychoanalysts are exceptional people (1968:531). Instead, she refers to the description given by Fliess of the psychoanalyst as a person who, outside of his professional function, most often is an ordinary person with the strengths and weaknesses that all people have, but who in his work possesses specific talents: ". . . the analyst must make possible what rightly seems impossible, because it is actually impossible for the average person, and must do so by becoming a very exceptional person during his work with the patient. To this end he will have to acquire a 'work-ego'" . . . (Fliess 1942:221).

I can imagine that many persons, belonging to a variety of professions, can recognize themselves here, in the way Fliess's "work-ego" is capable of realizing another and in many ways better professional ego than the one that appears to others in everyday relationships and commitments. We are not speaking here of "false selves" or playacting. Rather, it has to do with the capacity to do one's utmost within limited—and surely also limiting—frameworks without having to expose one's own desire or allowing the capriciousness of life to enter the scene.

Fliess's view is sobering in that it distances itself from the expansive and pedantic demands of the catalogues of virtue. To the merits of his concept belongs the fact that he neither defines nor fills the work-ego with any specific content. It is, after all, almost impossible to enumerate the analyst's wished-for qualities without slipping into the commonsensical tone of the catalogues of virtue.

To some extent this whole thing has to do with how we understand the nature of the selection process. Do we believe that we are sorting out the most gifted and suitable individuals, or do we restrict ourselves and avoid those we think are unsuitable or even detrimental to their patients? Van Der Leeuw writes: "Psycho-analysis is more and more being regarded as a method, a technique like any other, which the psychiatrist should be able to learn and to apply. Owing to this state of affairs selection is directed rather to exclusion of the unsuitable than to selection of the most suitable candidates" (1962:277). Professionalism's search for the averagely normal and suitable individual rather than the exceptionally talented person is strengthened by a reality in which it is so obviously difficult to formulate and agree on positive criteria.

In the above quote, van der Leeuw is judging the conditions prevailing in Europe at the beginning of the sixties; we must not presuppose that what he says is valid everywhere and always.[3] But, to the extent that his description is correct, it also makes any catalogues of virtues quite superfluous, for to avoid the unsuited applicants means that all we need is a set of criteria defining their unsuitability. Judging from what I have heard from different societies and differing persuasions, the usual list will contain the following items: psychosis, severe neurosis, perversions, manifest homosexuality, psychopathic character disorder, and asocial acting out (see Wallerstein 1978:487). One does indeed get the impression that it is felt to be much easier to intuitively recognize and define unwanted qualities than the ones that are valued (Dorn 1969:247).[4]

Here we touch upon the paradox of the professional versus the gifted analyst. The persistent wish to define what a psychoanalyst is or is expected to be is, of course, the expression of how the tendency to professionalization requires that one with some precision can select those suited or at least avoid the unsuitable ones. But the notorious difficulty—not to say impossibility—of succeeding in this leaves a vague and somewhat mysterious image of the analyst, which once again seems to engender in fantasy the so-beloved conception of the analyst as an exceptionally gifted person. And thus the circle is completed, and once again we will start listing required qualities.

Is it not precisely that fantasy that shows itself in the nostalgic return of the complaint that the individualistic, interested, curious, and creative personality of the first epoch is becoming more scarce, and that those who now take an interest in our practice are increasingly "normal" and averagely exemplary? This is not seldom mentioned as an effect of the fact that analysis has been granted social recognition and has acquired professional status. Knight illustrates this development from an unexpected point of view: "The convention cocktail parties and dinner dances which are regular program items today were unknown a decade and more ago. This 'normalizing' of the composition of the membership is an interesting and perhaps a significant phenomenon in the development of psychoanalysis in [the United States]" (1953:218).

In a considerably less jocular tone Smirnoff (1980) groups candidates into three rather coarse categories: (1) the insecure and passive ones who swallow concepts and theory without assimilating them and use them at a low and pragmatic level; (2) the conscientious ones who work hard, but will often disappoint us through their rigidity and lack of imagination; and (3) the curious, passionate, and nonconformist ones who every now and then are truly original but find it difficult to adapt to the discipline of organized training.

Bird writes rather revealingly that it is in fact just these "normal, stable, attractive and essentially nonscientific [candidates that are] needed as the core of a profession." And despite the fact that they often are mediocre, relatively unanalyzable, and seldom really good clinicians, "these 'normal characters' are rarely dropped from training but instead are nursed through at the cost of much faculty time and are finally graduated" (Bird 1968:515).[5] Therefore the artist, the philosopher, or the creative talent is a rare encounter within the professional team—too often being a bit too jumbled and unpredictable in a way that makes them a risk to the reputation of the profession. Professionalism rewards normality.

Among older and established psychoanalysts there seems to be a widespread dissatisfaction with the quality of younger colleagues: "With an increase in the number of psychoanalysts and institutes, a degree of mediocrity is creeping upon us" (Aarons 1982–1983:681).[6] And there may be something to the claim that the interplay between the professional institution and its team works to strengthen the position of those who are dependable and effective at the expense of those who are odd and at best perhaps creative. Bak points out that the creative personalities "with their manifold deviations, may be diffident about their acceptance, or even so repelled by having to run the gauntlet of admission procedures that they do not apply to us at all" (1970:13).

Usually, though, it is maintained that the question of the normal and "smoothly" symptom-free candidate touches upon something considerably more serious than the mere risk that the really gifted will never be admitted or that one might become bored in the company of colleagues. It has to do with the danger of letting the so-called normopaths, "as if" personalities, or those with a psychopathic character structure pass the controls of the selection system. It is, after all, one of the normopath's defining characteristics that he (or she) has developed a special talent for convincing the world around him that he is normal. When it comes to the normopath in training analysis it is not uncommon that he is described as firmly identifying with the training analyst, as if to thereby secure yet another aspect of the façade of normalcy. Torras De Beà presents the somewhat unusual idea that the real risk is not that these "normopaths" or "as if" personalities could possibly gain entrance to the training system because they can so easily make themselves inconspicuous, but because in fact they are all too well "in tune with training itself" (1992:161).

There is, of course, a kernel of truth in all these fears: the risk that one should admit someone who is clearly unsuitable or even deleterious to patients is a reality. But, just as one should critically assess the reasonableness in the concept of a steadily growing mediocrity among psychoanalysts it must also be asked whether the so often repeated fear of the psychopath possibly has to do with a figment of imagination and a paranoization of the social field.

A component of this paranoid structure—what I call "the psychoanalytic superego complex"—will be discussed in the chapter to follow. I mention it here because it is at least in part related to the process of selection. As we have seen, the primary requests are psychological characteristics and character traits. The most common practice is to subject the applicants to one or several more or less investigative interviews. The methods used for these interviews are most probably as varied as is the total group of interviewers, but it does seem that when the outcome of these encounters is to be assessed, the result is always the same: "Each meeting is a clinical conference in advanced psychopathology" (Eisendorfer 1959:374). The selection committees carry a great responsibility, both toward those colleagues who will analyze, supervise, and educate the candidates and one day also receive them as fellow analysts, and—this is of course the crucial point—toward future analysands whose human vulnerability, time, and even money must be protected from landing in the hands of analysts who simply are not suited for the job.

One should not (as many, and most probably analysts them-selves, seem to imagine) feel sure that psychoanalysts are better judges of character than others; it is, after all, not that for which they have been trained and it is not that with which they deal in their everyday work. But when they are asked to make a judg-ment they will, of course, utilize the very instruments at hand: a diagnostic apparatus and a clinical language created for interpret-ing and speaking of a profound experience with persons in men-tal distress. This is how the selection process turns into "advanced psychopathology"—and unfortunately also perhaps the first step in a sort of mental divestiture that will continue all through the training process and finally manifest itself in the form of institu-tionalized paranoia.

Now there is one criterion for suitability that is mentioned by many, but that does not really fit on the scale between virtue and straightforward unsuitability due to psychopathology, but that rather concerns itself with a certain kind of experience. Greenacre writes that a degree of neurosis is unavoidable among applicants and that it is not a sufficient ground for rejection. On the contrary, if it can be handled through a personal analysis it can even be an asset (1961:45). To those who emphasize this dimension it is taken for granted that the analyst should have experienced a true need for help and found it in his or her personal analysis: "A psycho-logically average, unremarkably healthy person will not do. The analyst-to-be needs to be to some extent disturbed and then to be successfully analysed" (Parsons 1984:457).

On the basis of such a criterion one will perhaps not select the exceptionally gifted, but on the other hand neither will one se-lect those who can be sorted out with the help of virtue catalogues or those who shine with their exemplary normality. It may well be asked whether the analytical training systems should take any interest at all in those who have not sought analysis because of a personal need. The capacity to encounter and handle one's neu-rotic suffering is not only an indication of the degree of humility and maturity we can expect of anyone who is to help others, but also a form of schooling within a world of experience from which he who seeks analytic treatment directs his cry for help. The name of that school is life itself and it is much more encompassing than the analytic training institution and, luckily, completely beyond its control. Heimann quotes the words of a colleague—Solms— saying: "After all, no matter how sophisticated our concepts of ego psychology have become, what we really expect in a psycho- analytic candidate is that he should have a good heart and that he should have gone through some suffering without denying it" (1968:537).

Leo Stone writes:

> I know of no adequate rational motivation for turning to analysis . . . other than the hope for relief of personal suffer- ing. . . . With regard to the training analysis, any colleague of some experience knows that its distinction from therapy is essentially fictive. It is usually a prolonged therapeutic analysis in which the professional aspiration is a special and complicating condition; the training aspect is an incidental by-product. [1975:353]

Stone adds the very pertinent comment that "only the hope for help . . . will motivate an individual to expose those elements in his personality which permit true analytic process and which can at times constitute genuine contributions to analytic science" (354).

The fact that "selection for psychoanalytic training means selection without a clear description of the concept of a 'good analyst' and without the possibility of evaluating the selection process" (Kappelle 1996:1214) together with the insight that we lack any form of objective instrument for prognostication, is still not the same as saying that the work of selection is meaningless and that the application system should be abolished. Even if the lack of reliable instruments is as topical today as it was in the fif- ties when we started considering the problems involved, and it still worries some that on the whole we act without really know- ing how and why, at least *some* kind of selection is indispensable— at least as long as psychoanalysis lives on within the institutional forms of the third epoch. I have the impression that there is a justified trust in the intuitive skillfulness which, despite all, makes it better to have a personally and psychologically oriented selection procedure rather than simple admission based upon formal merits, test results, or other "objective" data.[7] One must keep in mind that it is not merely a question of a "diagnosis" but also of a "prognosis"—the members of the selection committee must assess what they believe about the applicant's capacity to profit by the training analysis he is to embark upon.

DIDACTIC ANALYSIS, TRAINING ANALYSIS, PERSONAL ANALYSIS

[I]n listening to you here, I also got the impression that
my colleagues who first advocated the introduction of
training analysis at the Marienbad Congress—if they
had known of all the dangers, of the positive and negative transferences, and splits and hates, etc.—would
probably never have advocated it! They would have
said, "Let them be as they are!"
—A. Freud 1983:259

Since we lack any consensus on what it is that makes a
good analyst . . . we also lack consensus as to what the
training analysis should bring about.
—J. Cremerius 1987:1077–1078

From a medical viewpoint psychoanalysis is probably unique in that whomever is to conduct its method of treatment must first himself undergo it. To critics and skeptics this has been the target for sarcasms like "Who has ever heard of a coronary surgeon having to undergo a bypass operation as a part of his training?"

The indispensability of a personal analysis was clearly realized soon after Freud had developed the psychoanalytic method. Precisely because the analyst's field of work deals with the unconscious of another human being and that his own unconscious to such a great extent is an instrument for his work, he must be well acquainted with its workings in a way that far surpasses any self-knowledge we expect from one another in everyday social intercourse.

This state of affairs has contributed to the personal analysis—most commonly known as "training analysis"—traditionally being regarded as the most decisive aspect of the training. Thus, all the conceivable issues concerning the aims, the length, technique, reportability, the choice and qualifications of training analysts, its drawbacks and perils, and so forth have always been a center of focus.

In what follows I will attempt an investigation of training analysis based upon what I would like to designate as its four fundamental functions: (1) the therapeutic aim; (2) selection; (3) the transmission of an experience; and (4) the normalization of the analyst. Besides being guided by various explicit aims or intentions, these functions are intersected with hidden and not seldom unconscious purposes and structural effects that collaborate to form an invisible or tacit aspect of the training system. The order in which these functions follow does not mirror any intended ranking of their respective import, but simply follows basic considerations of representability.

The Therapeutic Aim

Balint (1954) enumerated five periods in the history of training analyses. During the first—the "period of instruction"—the task consisted mainly of a form of self-analysis on the basis of good knowledge of Freud's writings. The limitations to this were soon to be discovered and the "period of demonstration" was inaugurated. As is clear from the designation itself, now the aim of analysis was to display, through experience, the analytic method, convey to the candidate a conviction concerning the existence and importance of the unconscious, and to some extent convey a degree of insight intended to eradicate so-called blind spots.[8] As we have already seen, most often these "analyses" didn't last much more than a couple of weeks or at most a couple of months. These two initial periods passed practically without any discussion.

Only with the third period did "analysis proper" become a part of the regular curriculum. One might think that the beginning of this period would coincide with the Berlin Institute and the introduction of its training system, but that is not how Balint views things. And, reminding ourselves of what still, in 1930, could be written—with formulations like the aim of a didactic analysis (*Lehranalyse*) being to "refin[e] the future analyst's mental capacities" or "enrich the personality" (DpG 1930:59)—it is clear that at least during the first ten years of the Berlin Institute the view of training analysis did not conform with what today would be regarded as "psychoanalysis proper." Despite that, at the seventh congress in Berlin in 1922, it had already been decided that only those who had undergone a treatment with an analyst connected with the IPA were to be allowed to practice psychoanalysis and partake in theoretical seminars.[9]

At the same time, the idea was maintained that *didactic analysis did not need to be as "deep" or thoroughgoing as a therapeutic analysis*. This conception differs with abundant clarity from anything that would later be emphasized, namely the specific demands on any didactic analysis that it should be "deep" and precisely concentrate upon character formation.

Originally, the psychoanalytic method was conceived to be a form of treatment aimed at helping or relieving neurotic symptoms (i.e., such relatively well-defined manifestations as anxiety attacks, impotence, inhibitions, phobias, and so forth). Gradually, the method was to be developed to the point where it also included the analysis of character traits and even the character structure in its entirety. For a long time, though, character analysis was regarded as a particularly invasive measure.[10] A symptom is most often a disturbing part of the ego's world, a circumstance that makes it relatively easy for the analyst to establish an alliance with the analysand in his struggle against whatever it is that disturbs him. When it comes to character traits the situation is quite different; they are often felt to be an indispensable—albeit not always unproblematic—part of the ego, and therefore the analysand is more prone to defend them.[11] Therefore, character analysis will be directed more toward the analysand's defenses and his negative transference, which will make it both a more protracted and deep-going endeavor. The kind of analytic praxis regarded today as mainstream is basically oriented toward character analysis, even though one seldom encounters just that expression: character analysis has become so accepted that one simply says "analysis."

According to Balint's description the demand for "analysis proper" came about as a result of Ferenczi's critique against the demonstration model, and the changeover itself came only after protracted discussions and against considerable resistance. Ferenczi said that a training analysis must be as time-consuming and profound as any regular therapeutic analysis, and at the congress in Innsbruck in 1927 the ITC put forth the request that an analyst should be better analyzed than his analysands. Those who opposed this idea thought that character formation was the most valuable aspect of the personality and nothing to tinker with. Instead, it was necessary to be sure to protect and preserve the candidate's "personality or . . . character" (Kovács 1936: 349–350).

Balint states that this controversy was never really solved. Instead, it was forgotten in conjunction with the transition to the fourth period, during which time analysts paradoxically tried to live up to even more ambitious goals resulting in what Balint calls a "supertherapy." This was yet another idea of Ferenczi's invention. He writes that when we are speaking of the analyst himself a regular analysis is not sufficient, for he "must know and be in control of even the most recondite weaknesses of his own character; and this is impossible without a *fully completed analysis*" (Ferenczi 1928:84; my italics).

To use—like Balint does—Freud's slightly ironic formulations to characterize this level of ambition, we could say that "what we are asking is whether the analyst has had such a far-reaching influence on the patient that no further change could be expected to take place in him if his analysis were continued.

It is as though it were possible by means of analysis to attain a level of absolute psychical normality" (Freud 1937:219–220). Freud warns his readers not to be overly zealous when it comes to the analyses of future analysts. He writes that for practical reasons they can only be short and incomplete (although he does not explain why this should be so).[12] And, to balance any unrealistic expectations (for example, in the form of the notion of a supertherapy) he recommends recurrent reanalyses, perhaps every fifth year or so. Thus, the analyst's analysis must be an interminable one (249).

Despite Glover ten years earlier having already pointed out the dangers inherent in any conception of "the perfectly analyzed analyst" (1927)—and this possibly as a reply to Ferenczi—Freud's ironical skepticism did not suffice to avert a development where since the middle of the thirties training analyses the world over were to become evermore protracted—to the point, writes Balint some twenty years later, that "to-day I think it is fair to say that nobody has any idea how long a training analysis should or does last" (1954:158).

Balint finishes his periodization with a fifth era, where the training analyses are regarded as a kind of "research." He indicates that this period has been entered upon at the time when he writes his article, but does not really define what he means. Weigert's interpretation of Balint's expression makes of it a matter of candidates seeking analysis not so much from a personal need, but because they are driven by a research interest and professional ambitions, which will make these analyses more didactic rather than straightforwardly therapeutic. Weigert is enthusiastic about Balint's category and says: "It seems important to me that we not only name training analysis 'research analysis,' but that we accept the spirit of research" (Weigert 1955:639).

Even though the idea of training analysis as a form of "research" has scarcely won any acceptance, Balint's distinction between "supertherapy" and "research analysis" does point toward the important issue of whether and to what extent a training analysis differs from a "regular, therapeutic" one.

It seems as if the prewar generation of psychoanalysts preferred not to perceive any difference between training analysis and "regular, therapeutic" analysis. Hanns Sachs, who was the first appointed training analyst, writes in an article where he summarizes a life of work that "I have found the difference between the analyses of training candidates and of neurotic patients negligible" (Sachs 1947:158). Maxwell Gitelson, belonging to a later generation of analysts, writes that "we can no longer make a valid distinction between therapeutic analysis and training analysis" (1948:205).

As we have seen, in Balint's discussion on differences, most contributions concerned the high demands that must be placed upon the analyst. Even if it is true that Freud viewed the expectations lying behind such demands with a certain skepticism, the idea that a training analysis must go further and deeper has been difficult to eradicate. Sacha Nacht writes, for example, that "to penetrate into the unconscious as deeply as possible is a task still more essential in a training analysis than in a therapeutic one" (1954:253).[13] On the whole, Balint's observation consists in the fact that *all modern training institutes are—and remain—deeply influenced by the idea of supertherapy*. I would go one step further and say that supertherapy is the very ideal for training analysis that has prevailed and still prevails during the third epoch of the psychoanalytic institution—an ideal which, according to Greenacre, merely betrays a lack of trust within psychoanalytic institutes in their own selection processes (1961:41).

The demand for supertherapy in the form of character analysis or deep investigations into the unconscious[14] has a different background than that for analytic excellence. Grete Bibring writes that "our selection of candidates is bound to lead to the prevalence of character-analyses" (1954:169). The inevitability here has more to do with the fact that "[i]n a therapeutic analysis the patient asks the analyst to restore his health. In a training analysis the analytic Society briefs the analyst to introduce the candidate to the career he has chosen" (Heimann 1954:163). The future candidate simply has a different *motive* for embarking upon an analysis.

When the wish to rid oneself of some personal problem or impediment is only second in priority it is still to be expected that the processes of resistance and defense will be just as prominent as in a regular analysis, albeit perhaps somewhat less dramatic. American findings suggest that "regular, therapeutic" training analyses are often emotionally "cooler" than regular analyses (Shapiro 1976:34), a phenomenon that might just depend on the fact that so many personal analyses are undertaken for purely professional reasons, which is to say, in Balint's words, that they tend to become "research analyses."[15] To this difficulty also belongs what Gitelson points out, namely that the "normality" that a prospective candidate presents is a kind of symptom with its specific rewards—not in the least in the form of social acceptance (1954:179–180). So even if the candidate's analysis is a "regular, therapeutic" character analysis, this character may—due to the surrounding conditions—turn out to be particularly difficult to access for analytical investigation.[16]

As part of the applicant's/candidate's pathology belongs the important but evasive issue concerning his wish to become a psychoanalyst. In the letter of invitation to an IPA conference, "Clinical Approaches to the Termination of the Training Analysis," in Santiago, Chile, in the summer of 1999, two interesting questions were raised: "Should the desire to become an analyst be viewed as a symptom in need of analysis?" and "When a candidate decides not to become a psychoanalyst, should this be regarded as a good outcome of the analysis?" These are questions that touch upon something that has always been a preoccupation of those who have reflected upon the conditions for training since the birth of the psychoanalytic institution.

Of course, there is always good reason to investigate the issue—to the extent that this is possible. It is evident that everyone is not suited for the task, but one might well ask whether such a choice—analytically a symptom *strictu sensu*, that is to say a dynamic compromise—would allow for its being analyzed in any "complete" sense. Isn't it rather that the desire behind the wish to become a psychoanalyst will only unfold during the course of a whole professional life as we discover what it is in the psycho-analytical experience that gives us joy and pleasure?[17] And if we indeed stick to the idea that the wish to become an analyst is some-thing to be completely illuminated in the training analysis, would the paradoxical risk then be that "[i]f we were able to analyse [the wish to be an analyst] thoroughly, would that not make an end of further training?" (Nielsen 1954:248).

Selection and Evaluation

Apart from whatever differences there may be between "or-dinary," therapeutic analyses and training analyses when it comes to depth, intensity, goals, and so forth, there is one dissimilarity that more directly concerns the demands posed by the training institute. As we have seen, the praxis of the Berlin Institute was not to accept candidates for training before they had undergone a "trial analysis," after which the training analyst would report to the Institute his evaluation of the applicant's suitability for embarking upon the training proper and ultimately having pa-tients in treatment.

During a period of intervening events (see below under "The Supervised Cases") this way of using training analysis as an in-strument for selection was gradually abandoned and replaced with a procedure that in many ways was still similar. I say "similar," for in fact this new procedure—where candidates are accepted for training while at the same time the training analyst is expected to advise the institute against further training if the candidate shows serious signs of unsuitability—is really nothing other than a variation of the trial analyses of the first epoch.[18] Now the can-didate was selected for training after being individually evaluated, but the training analyst had to give his approval before the can-didate started attending theoretical seminars or began with su-pervised cases. Ultimately, the training analyst was to give his opinion of the candidate when the latter was to graduate and become a certified psychoanalyst.

Lewin and Ross (1960) coined the term *syncretism* to designate the specific problems that will follow from such a system. In the *Oxford English Dictionary* the word is defined as the "attempted union or reconciliation of diverse or opposite tenets or practices, esp. in philosophy or religion." In the case of psychoanalysis, syncretism has to do with the contradictory attempt on the one hand to offer a genuine experience of a psychoanalysis, with its exclusive intimacy and the explicit or implicit promise of absolute confidentiality, and on the other to introduce didactic and controlling elements by which the analyst is expected to be the judge of his analysand and report on the basis of what has been said in confidence. It should be no surprise that training analyses during discussions in the fifties and sixties so often are spoken of as incomplete or even, for the most part, failures.

What, then, would a defense sound like for such a burdensome compromise between therapeutic interests and didactic intentions? One of the more detailed instances appears in an article by Calef and Weinshel in 1973. Initially it is suggested that "the therapeutic results of the training analysis are not anywhere as dismal as many analysts have assumed" (p. 715; see also Shapiro 1976). The authors continue by saying that the majority of discussants on this issue have too loosely equated reporting as such with a breach of confidentiality. They believe that reporting cannot essentially be distinguished from the everyday task whereby the analyst assesses the analysand's progress. They also underscore the absurdity of a training institute certifying a candidate solely on the basis of judgments coming from teachers and supervisors: the decisive criterion must be the candidate's analyzability.[19] Their conclusive argument betrays a tangible fear of what would happen if the training analyst/institute were to give up controlling power:

All candidates in analysis come into that situation with the fears and fantasies of having certain defects and deficiencies relating to their capacity to be analyzed and to being analysts, and of having these defects and deficiencies exposed. Obviously, these fears have much more complex and archaic roots; but in the immediate analytic situation they foster certain resistances, among which are those which relate to reporting. These resistances and their underlying fantasies and conflicts cannot be resolved merely by promising not to report. On the contrary, such a pact might tend to enhance the resistances and interfere with their ultimate resolution. [725]

Among the issues on which a training analyst might report, Fleming and Weiss mention: "Is there a firm working alliance?", "Is the candidate able to associate freely?", "What is the stage of transference development?", "Has the transference meaning of matriculation been worked on in the analysis?", "How strong a defence is acting out with resistance against analysing it?", "How likely is the presence of a supervisor to interfere with analysing?" (1978:38).

The fact that Lewin and Ross made the syncretistic dilemma visible by putting a label on it seems to have urged on a discussion that surely would have taken place in any case, albeit perhaps without the same speed and force. Particularly in the United States, the sixties and seventies witnessed an animated debate between the increasingly frequent critical voices and the equally persevering defenders of the reporting system. One of the crucial publications coming from the critical camp was Kairys's "The Training Analysis—A Critical Review of the Literature and a Controversial Proposal" (1964), an article that was to become almost the foundation for all subsequent discussion, whether one was critical of the reporting system or defended it.[20]

Kairys's article, which in part is a commentary upon what up to then had been published concerning the problems of training analyses, starts by mentioning what Balint had been able to establish sixteen years earlier, namely, that the number of texts dealing with training and training analysis is conspicuously small. Both authors suggest that this is the result of suppression and censorship. Taking as his point of departure the concept of syncretism, Kairys mentions the specific transference problems encumbering the training analyses: they are simply not as successful as the ordinary psychoanalytic treatments. For that reason many analysts suffer unresolved infantile attitudes and transferential fixations in a way that will hamper both their relationship with the surrounding world and with the analytic profession.

For a favorable analytic process to come into being, there must be room for a transference to evolve that is sufficiently uncontaminated by real factors, such as knowledge of the analyst's person or by his real intervention in the analysand's life. A candidate's feeling that his analyst is possibly judging him cannot be ascribed only to transference factors; within an institute that encourages its training analysts to report on "their" candidates, that is most probably also a correct perception. In short: within the reporting system the analyst performs precisely those kinds of actions that the professional ethic otherwise condemns on good grounds, as it deems them to be antitherapeutic and detrimental.[21]

The syncretistic dilemma leads to a situation where no candidate can fully trust his training analyst, and when it comes to the extent of damages issuing from the reporting system, Kairys's impression is that they are very widespread. There were no attempts to measure these deleterious effects with statistical methods at the time of Kairys's article, nor are there any today.[22]

It is not part of the analyst's task to judge his analysand, however considerately and discreetly this may be done. His obligation is to be present for an *encounter* with the analysand, which is something quite different. To put it briefly, there is no foundation whatsoever for the expectation that the training analyst would be superior in judging the candidate as compared with others in his environment (cf. Lifschutz 1976:57). It is certainly true that an analyst knows a lot concerning his analysand, but it is equally true that he is involved, engaged in, and to some extent inevitably identified with his analysand (more on this under the rubric "A State within the State" in Chapter 5). It is therefore in the nature of things that as an evaluator the analyst is always biased.

Kairys's proposal consisted of the simple but at that time controversial recommendation to "divorce the training analysis completely from the rest of the student's training" (Kairys 1964:506). The candidate would still undergo a training analysis with a training analyst, but the latter would respect exactly the same rules of discretion and confidentiality that guide other analyses, and under no circumstances would he discuss the candidate's analytic progress with the committees of the institute. All necessary information underlying a decision to graduate or not graduate a candidate would come from seminar teachers and supervisors.[23,24]

The decisive turn in the discussions on reporting and nonreporting came during the seventies, when practically all psychoanalytic institutes around the world gradually accepted the model that proposed a total division between training analysis and all other educational demands. Judging from various suggestions in the literature, this did not always change at once, and in certain cases a system remained in which those training analysts who so wished could refrain from reporting while others would continue with the old way of doing things (see, for example, McLaughlin 1973). During the eighties, however, the nonreporting system seems to have become almost ubiquitous.[25]

When the training analyst's obligation to report disappeared from most institutes, a gradual transition took place beginning in the seventies, when the view that the training analysis should be regarded as the central element of the training was given up and in its stead greater emphasis was placed on the candidate's experience of conducting psychoanalysis under supervision.[26]

It is only after this shift—when it is no longer a didactic factor—that one can really speak of a "personal analysis." In essence, it is to be only therapeutic and restricted to being merely a basic requirement for graduating as a psychoanalyst.[27]

With these changes a limited but immensely important step was taken toward increasing candidates' autonomous self-evaluation—or their analytical ego-strength, to use the language of Fliess and Balint. When control is lifted from the training analysis the candidate is given clearer authority to judge on the basis of his own insights whether he is worthy of or suitable for the task of being a psychoanalyst (see G. Bibring 1954:173; McLaughlin 1973:707).

The Transmission of an Experience

The transmission of an experience was an idea originally formulated by Ferenczi and Rank in 1924. When it comes to the effects of a training analysis one often speaks of identification processes, especially the candidate's identification with his analyst: "Identification is the central mechanism in all programs of education" (Arlow 1972:560); "The educational goal in training psychoanalysts is to foster that kind of identification which is stable, secure, and resistant to regressive reinvolvement in conflict" (563).

Identification is not a unitary concept, but rather a collective term to designate a number of differing processes, and possibly not even the best one in this connection. Laplanche and Pontalis define identification as a "psychological process whereby the subject assimilates an aspect, property or attribute of the other and is transformed, wholly or partially, after the model the other provides. It is by means of a series of identifications that the personality is constituted and specified" (1967:205). Evident from this theoretically loose formulation identification is—and seems to remain—a complex psychoanalytic concept that in fact might better be replaced with a set of more differentiated concepts. (One area where the term certainly does apply, however, in the sense of emulating the other by choosing that person as one's model, is the narcissistic tie that perhaps inevitably will arise between the training analyst and the candidate.[28] This issue is discussed below under the rubric "A State within the State" in Chapter 5.)

The Internalization of the Analyst's Function

The one single experience with the greatest importance for the analyst's conception of the analytical task, for his analytical "style," and perhaps also for his relationship to the analytical community is his personal analysis (or analyses). Apart from the experience of being an analysand, assimilation of the experience of being an analyst takes place. That should be the case in all analyses, but it is never so decisive as when the analysand one day is to become an analyst himself.

Instead of the term "identification," a concept for a process where the traits and personality of the other are to be emulated, I prefer to speak of *internalization*, a process where inter-subjective relationships are absorbed and transformed into subjective structures. Let me illustrate: beyond the self-evident demand that the caregiver must adapt to the needs of the infant, it is also inevitable that the newborn will "capture" the care-giving environment's specific ways of functioning—its rhythms, whims, and fluctuating capacity for care. The psychoanalytic experience demonstrates—not least through the phenomenon of transference—that assimilation of that kind is not merely reactive and passive, but that it will later surface as a disposition to exercise the same kind of functions as the subject himself once encountered. A classic in that vein is, for example, the belated but nevertheless horrifying discovery that in our parental function we will reproduce a number of precisely those traits we once promised ourselves never to subject our own children to. Despite our best intentions to the opposite, there are apparently forces that tend to make us become like our parents.

Theoretically this may not be elaborated very well, but it is important to point out how the analytical candidate absorbs his own analyst's manner of being together with him: such things as the analyst's way of listening, his patterns when it comes to hold-ing back or intervening, how he sits and moves in his chair, how he prepares and formulates his interventions, his way of making use of humor, his inventiveness, how he shows respect and con-sideration, his ways of modulating his voice to convey (or disguise) warmth, understanding, sympathy, confusion, irritation, disap-proval, disgust, indignation, and whether he is characterologically sentimental or unsentimental.[29]

The training analyst thus offers a personally colored emotional and affective milieu that leaves an impression on the candidate's *habitus*, his way of being in the world and of relating to it. In this expectation also dwells the above-mentioned possibility that he may turn out to be what he once may have wished not to be. Conversely, there is also the possibility—without effort, I would almost say without the *work* of identification—of being precisely that which one has encountered but did not believe oneself capable of. *That* is what I would call the assimilation of the analyst's style. This *habitus* is comparable to what Robert Fliess speaks of (and was dealt with above) when he describes the analyst as a person who is an ordinary human being outside his professional function, but who in his work "must make possible what rightly seems impossible, because it is actually impossible for the average person, and must do so by becoming a very exceptional person during his work with the patient. To this end he will have to acquire a 'work-ego' . . ." (1942:221).[30]

The "work-ego" actualizes a different and in many ways better professional ego than what the analyst otherwise will demonstrate in his everyday dealings with the world. This is not a question of emulation or of seeking to be this or that. The acquisition of a work-ego rests, among other factors, upon precisely the absorption of a "style," a manner of being a psychoanalyst, which is transmitted via one's own analyst. Regretfully, I must make the observation that this will be valid both when it comes to good relations between analysand and training analyst and when it comes to those who are unsound and corrupt. It should come as no surprise that an inferior or defective training analysis will tend to foster a weak analyst.

It is more or less well known that one cannot stray far from the analytical style one once has acquired. To become a Kleinian analyst it will not suffice to read Klein and Kleinian theory: one has to have felt the Kleinian experience on one's own skin, as it were. I myself have made the same discovery when attempting to appropriate Lacanian technique. Despite excellent supervision it would not work because I lacked the necessary experience of a clinical situation structured in accordance with Lacanian principles.[31]

Insight into the Conditions of the Analytic Process

The analytic process is a wide spectrum of events that are also difficult to wholly distinguish from what has been discussed under the above rubric. There really is no way to know what psychoanalysis is all about other than by way of personal experience. The personal analysis prepares the candidate for what he will be in search of later on while working with his own supervised cases.

The decisive experience in this connection is becoming acquainted with the transference. The matrix of transference is, as I tried to demonstrate in Chapter 2, the central playground for the intersubjectivity of the analytical dyad. Mere study of the literature will not bring about an understanding of what that kind of interaction truly is about—at least not without severe misconceptions.

The matrix of transference forms a specific and peculiar psychic space enveloping analyst and analysand. To recognize this very special scene and to be able to foster the development of something similar in his own work, the candidate must have had the experience and be rather well seasoned to its characteristic atmosphere.

Having himself once been privy to the analytical situation will lay the foundations for the candidate's subsequent capacity to understand his analysand's position. Thus he is offered the opportunity to really grasp that the analysand is a fellow being in distress, with deep expectations aimed at the candidate and their joint work of being helped. That seems to be one of the most difficult lessons to be learned during analytical training, which to my mind makes it so much more urgent that the candidate once actually did seek analysis out of personal need and not for mere professional reasons.

With sympathy for the analysand's plight comes such things as tact and regard. Even if psychoanalytical practice on good grounds does not adhere to the generally accepted ethic of care of our Judaeo-Christian culture, expressions of compassion and consideration are in no way excluded, and here there is a legacy for the candidate to put to good use as, in gratitude for the reception he once enjoyed from his own analyst, he is able to offer his analysands something similar.

In Chapter 2 I mentioned faith in the Other as an essential element in the analytical attitude. I described this faith in terms of insight into and acceptance of the fact that the Other essentially escapes my knowledge and my wish to objectify him. Faith in the Other rests upon a horizon of expectation; it is the sustained hope of a coming encounter with the analysand within the frame of the matrix of transference.

So, much more than a form of technical dexterity, faith in the Other is a gift of sorts bequeathed in silence, a composure in not always being in the know, which makes it possible for the candidate to *await the Other* rather than reach closure by objectivating him on the basis of the categories of his knowledge. Here, then, we can identify that process whereby he who has been subjected to a function in his turn may exercise it in relation to another.

I believe that the acquisition of the "finer" aspects of the psychoanalytic method comes about through precisely those invisible and pedagogically tacit forms of transmission of the requested attitude toward the analysand and the task itself. Therein lies one of the most central functions of the personal analysis.

To Become a Keeper in the Service of the Analytical Setting

If one who is liberated from any ideas of psychological content and medically founded conceptions of treatment and cure were to ascertain what psychoanalytical training really wants to accomplish, I would say that its goal is to make of the candidate *a skillful keeper of the analytical setting*. In the *Oxford English Dictionary* "keeper" is defined as "one who guards, protects, or preserves; . . . one to whom the care and preservation of any thing is committed." If there is anything that embodies the ethos of the psychoanalytic experience, it would not only be the analyst's way of keeping watch over the setting, but also his tending it so that the best preconditions for analytical work in the service of the analysand will always prevail. Without its strict setting, analytical work would rapidly deteriorate into benevolent helpfulness and moral treatment.[32]

To the central elements of the setting belong the following:

1. Every session starts and ends at the minutes agreed upon, usually 45 minutes to an hour; within those confines there is an atmosphere of "timelessness" and no termination date is decided in advance.
2. Clear instructions concerning costs and forms of payment are given.
3. There is a spatial arrangement where the analyst most often sits behind the analysand, who is lying on a couch. There is no eye contact.
4. The fundamental rule of psychoanalysis is observed, namely that the analysand speak freely of whatever is occupying his feelings and thoughts.
5. The analyst's neutrality is maintained, which, among other things, implies that he strives to supply the analysand with as little knowledge as possible concerning his own person, his views, and his desire.
6. There is incorruptible confidentiality on the part of the analyst.

Enumerated like this, the elements of the setting may seem to be a list of rules that are simple to follow. And so it may be at times, but what is truly essential to underscore in this connection is *how the handling of the setting in the encounter between the candidate and his analyst can be transmitted as the implicit ethic of the analytical dialogue*—in other words, as the very opposite of the traditional deontology so often handed out in the set of rules of professional ethics (see note 34 to Chapter 5): "The setting . . . depends not only on technique, but again on the personality of the psychoanalyst"

(Torras de Beà 1992:160). It is then possible to speak of the keeping of the setting as an expression of the analyst's character or attitude. Cultivated in that fashion, the setting "holds" the analytical relation and guarantees that it will be a creative space for the analysand and not an opportunity for the analyst to (unconsciously) appropriate for himself emotional or other benefits.[33]

To become a skillful keeper of the analytical setting is, in other words, an ethical task, and conscientiousness in this sphere has permeated analytical training ever since its birth. Likewise, the maintenance and strengthening of this ethic is one of the fundamental motives for analysts to devote themselves to such a high degree to professional encounters in their societies, at seminars, and at congresses. There is a strong need to guard the analytical attitude against erosive influences provided by the surrounding world.

But as the ethical core of the aim to create a keeper of the analytical setting will only seldom be spoken of in terms of an ethical good, but more often in terms of "analytic technique," the institutional forms for transmitting the function of the setting rather contribute to the "normalization" of the analyst, and the handling of the setting tends to become an issue having to do with "correct or orthodox procedures" rather than being the expression of the analyst's autonomy and maturity.

The Normalization of the Analyst

To travesty an old expression[34] we might say that the normalization of the analyst has as its ultimate goal to produce an "average expectable psychoanalyst"—but, be it noted, not the statistically average analyst, or one who is acceptably "normal" to the intended analysand. No, the orderer is in this case the psychoanalytical community itself.

> When we give our pupils theoretical instruction in psychoanalysis, we can see how little impression we are making on them to begin with. They take the theories of analysis as coolly

as other abstractions with which they are nourished. A few of them may perhaps *wish* to be convinced, but there is not a trace of their being so. But we also require that everyone who wants to practise analysis on other people shall first himself submit to an analysis. It is only in the course of this [training analysis], when they actually experience as affecting their own person—or, rather, their own mind—the processes asserted by analysis, that they acquire the convictions by which they are later guided as analysts. [Freud 1926:198–199, italics in original]

"The normalization of the candidate" would, in this connection, imply the adaption of his ways of thinking about the psychoanalytical project, the unconscious and psychic conflict according to the norm, or that "conviction," as Freud says, that prevails within a certain group or school. The importance of "conviction" must not be underestimated, and "induction into the analytic movement, it seems, is not a matter of learning certain skills, but of absorbing certain values" (Frosch 1997:7). In other words, the target aimed at is a strong identification with the training analyst, or at least with his theory and/or his analytical technique: "We know that the general aim of all initiation rites is to force the candidate to identify himself with his initiator, to introject the initiator and his ideals, and to build up from these identifications a strong super-ego which will influence him all his life" (Balint 1948:167).

The most decisive moment in that process is the training analysis, that part of the candidate's training where he is the most susceptible to the authority of his mentors. One simple expression of this is that training institutes have traditionally required that the candidates' personal analyses always be with a training analyst belonging to the institute itself, even when there are other analysts available belonging to other societies that in other connections are regarded as equals. In most societies with well-defined groups it has been rather unusual that the supervisor and theoretical inclination chosen should belong to any group other than that of the training analyst (see Arlow 1982:12–13; Greenacre 1966).

One may say that "a training analysis . . . is inevitably influenced by strong pushes toward conformity and acceptance" (Richards 1997:122), but there are apparently stronger forces than mere adaptability at work here. Even more drastic than calling the process of normalization a rite of initiation is to say that it is a form of indoctrination, as does Kernberg: "Psychoanalytic education today is all too often conducted in an atmosphere of indoctrination rather than of open scientific exploration" (1986:799).

As to the "conviction" mentioned by Freud in the above quote, it may very well be true that "the analyst must be firmly persuaded in order to conduct good work" (Beland 1983:62). The question is what kind of persuasion is required. I believe that there is one and only one conviction that the presumptive candidate must bring with him as he looks for analytical training, and that is a strongly held belief that unconscious processes are the basis of all conscious mental action and that these processes influence our aims and actions in a way that will not let itself be wholly controlled by conscious rational deliberation (it must be stated, however, that conviction concerning the existence of the unconscious is not necessarily the same as being confirmed in one's beliefs as to specified unconscious contents).

I stated above that during the third epoch of the analytic institution the training institutes were deeply influenced by the idea of supertherapy. In the invitation to the IPA "Conference of Training Analysts" in Santiago, Chile, in 1999, the arrangers asked: "How are we to understand the prolonged duration of training analyses in our days?" Thomä writes: "One falls back on giving value to quantitative factors: the longer the better" (1993:30). In fact, the duration of training analyses seems to grow, and today in Germany the number of sessions is close to 1000, and in other countries it may be even higher than that (28). Training analyses conducted with five or six sessions per week during five, six years or even more—and which will have a total of up to 1,500 sessions—are no rarity (see, for example, Wallerstein 1978:494). Contributing to this protraction is the common demand that the training analysis should take place at least during some part of the time while the candidate conducts his supervised analyses.

> I have not noticed that the important contributions are made by analysts who went through ten years of personal analysis. I am sure I'll be forgiven if I don't substantiate my statements with names.
>
> —R. Bak 1970:16

Kleinian analyses are especially noted to be extraordinarily lengthy (see Greenacre 1961:41; Limentani 1986:238; Wallerstein 1978:490).[35] Whether the issue is clearly aired or not, the intention would be to imbue the candidate with a specific way of perceiving the processes of the unconscious: "in the Kleinian system the aim of the purification [from blind spots] is not to do away with the countertransference but to ensure that the analyst is open to a special kind of perception of the patient's unconscious" (Thomä 1993:31).[36] Robert Bak quotes Charlotte Babcock, who, in a report on training analysis writes of "a trend toward lengthy training analyses which in some instances had the deleterious effect of encouraging an unrealistic dependency in the candidate or an over-identification with his analyst" (1970:16).

> The personal analysis anyhow tends to infantilize the analysand temporarily and to a certain degree. When we incorporate it into a school system in which the student is treated as the object of abstract rules, this infantilism is intensified. When he has to stay in this atmosphere a long time it is made very difficult for him to see psychoanalysis for what it really is—a tool to strengthen one's intellectual, emotional, and social independence. [Bernfeld 1962:480]

As was discussed in Chapter 2 concerning theoretical work, it seems to be a rule that no psychoanalytic theories about man's "inner world" fit well with what we in our everyday self-reflection find within ourselves—especially, of course, if the work of theoretical assimilation has been shallow or neglected. For the analytical experience to become meaningful, the analysand must be able to identify with the language used by his analyst. This requires that the analyst manifest an authority conveying that he *knows* something that the analysand is still unaware of. Such a process takes more time the more the analyst's clinical imagery differs from the language of commonsense psychological knowledge. In a posthumously published paper of 1963, W. R. Bion mentions a patient who

> though aware of the approach of a car, walked out in front of it, was knocked down, and sustained minor injuries. This result was apparently quite unexpected. Many of his statements had prepared me to expect that he was dominated at the time of the event by the conviction that he was a puff of flatus. . . . I therefore said that he felt the car accident was a sexual intercourse between a puff of flatus and the car and its driver. He said he felt better and added he felt he was going mad. [Bion 1997:16–20]

Regardless of one's personal convictions as to the reasonableness of Bion's interpretational metaphorics in this instance, it would be quite evident to anyone that it would take some time to accept images such as these into one's own self-reflection. (And should the analysand in this case really have felt better—adding that he felt he might be going mad—this seeming paradox may have to do with his feeling that Bion made an honest attempt at understanding him, but that at the same time he was expected to ingest ideas that seemed rather mad.) It might be a good thing to discuss, more than seems to have been done, to what extent the analytical process is dependent upon the analysand's submission to the analyst's metaphors. In any case, when it comes to training analyses, it would seem to be a matter of course that the candidate's surrender to and even identification with the forms of self-reflection that are offered contribute to his "normalization" and gradual transformation into an acceptable colleague with the same language and convictions as the other members of the group he has chosen to be part of.

   The indoctrinating effect—even if it seldom is spoken of as such—is presumably a universal function in all psychoanalytic training and works like an aid in incorporating the candidate in the institutional superego system. A structurally similar result of what has just been mentioned was striven for by, for example, the British Society's Anna Freudians. Adam Limentani tells of how Anna Freud would point out that a good training analysis would be a guarantee that the candidate would never seek any other kind of help for personal problems in the future than psychoanalysis—an idea he himself takes for granted would be supported by most of his colleagues (Limentani 1992:133).

A common thought—or attempt at consolation, one might say—when it comes to the problems and imperfections connected with training analyses is the notion of *a second analysis*:

> There are experienced analysts in whose judgment personal analysis during training is so complicated or even deformed as to make it therapeutically almost valueless. In the opinion of some, the training analysis had best be accepted largely as a teaching situation, a truly didactic performance in which therapeutic goals are only secondary. A therapeutic analysis may then be sought at a later time according to the individual's awareness of unresolved problems as he discovers them in the course of his practice. Such a second analysis is then for one's self, in contrast to the first which was for training. [Greenacre 1966:559]

This idea has been so seductive to some that it has been proposed that a second analysis should be compulsory (Nacht 1954:253; see also Jones 1937:273). The issue is in no way a historical curiosity; one can come upon ardent advocates of a second analysis to this day.

Greben mentions a discussion with a colleague who had undergone a second analysis and who started out by talking about his training analysis: "I learned early on that there was a great deal I was not going to accomplish with him. However, my training was at stake, and I decided to get through it as quickly as I could. But now I've picked someone I can be more open with, and I'm getting a great deal more out of it" (1982–1983:665).[37] If the compulsory training analysis has been unsatisfactory it is, of course, quite natural that the analyst look for a second analysis, but it is appalling to think of the enormous waste of time, money, and engagement that would be the result of the training analysis systematically being regarded merely as a didactic undertaking (see Kairys 1964:505–506). And what would it then be? Would it at all be possible to regard it as psychoanalysis?

There is yet another aspect to the question of a second analysis. In some societies it used to be common practice that the candidate's analyst and supervisors would be appointed by the institute (see Greenacre 1966:547). Nowadays, however, the (prospective) candidate is usually allowed to choose whichever training analyst he wants to see. But, he who in naive openness once may have looked for help to solve personal problems will here meet with an initially invisible coercive force that may turn out to be rather painful when he finds out that analysis with someone who is not a training analyst will not be accepted by the institute and that he now must choose one from their list: "The institute *requires* an analysis, a reality situation interfering with independent inner wishes to be analyzed" (Dorn 1969:248). Not only may this be an enormous waste of time and money, but it is also a fact that "often the fate of these people is not a particularly happy one" (Thomä 1993:24, italics in original).

THE SUPERVISED CASES

Supervision as an educational technique is a very complicated matter. It involves all aspects of the pedagogical interaction. In some respects supervision differs not at all from the ordinary tutorial method of teaching. In other respects it resembles a clinical conference and at times it takes on the form, however briefly, of a didactic lecture.

—J. Arlow 1963:576

As we have seen in the previous chapter, the Berlin Institute developed a specific training function called "control analysis" (in more contemporary terminology one now speaks of supervised cases), the aim of which was a deepening of the experience of the practical procedures of psychoanalytic treatment that the candidate would have acquired during his training analysis. The control cases were thus regarded as a sort of supplement to the training analysis and the candidate's "treatment of patients is, so to speak, the touchstone by which we test the result of his own analysis" (Bibring 1937:372). (To the tasks allotted to the training analyst traditionally belong both the analysis of candidates and their supervision. In this section I will distinguish between these two functions by reserving the term "training analyst" for the former and "supervisor" for the latter.)

In our day the supervised cases constitute perhaps the central element of the tripartite model of training—at least when it comes to the evaluation of the candidate. The connection with the personal analysis is still present in that the candidate will be allowed to embark upon analytical work of his own only after having been evaluated by the institute, a test most often based on whether the candidate is deemed as having made sufficient "progress" in his personal development (i.e., in his own analysis) in whatever way that is done when lacking information from the training analyst. Supervision is most often conducted individually, even though group supervision does occur in some institutes.[38]

The requirements as to the number of supervised cases, their duration, frequency, and how often supervision should take place vary among different institutes and countries. The most prevalent requirement is three or four supervised cases—in some societies with the additional requisite that a certain number of them be concluded before matriculation. Sometimes there will be a demand of a minimal total number of sessions, or a minimal stretch of years conducting each treatment. When it comes to frequency, the most common demand is that the candidate see his analysands four or five times a week (usually for 45 or 50 minutes). Even though it deviates from official IPA policy, it is in some instances accepted to allow the supervised cases (as with the training analyses) to be conducted with only three sessions per week.[39] The requirements concerning the total length of these analyses may differ. How these requirements are codified vary to such an extent that it would be impossible to try to account for them in detail. On the whole, though, the sum of sessions in supervised cases before graduation seems to land somewhere between 500 and 1000.

Early in the development of the psychoanalytical institution candidates would be assigned by their institute to both training analysts and supervisors. They were not allowed to choose those persons who were to become so important to their personal and professional lives. The universally prevailing system today seems to be that the candidate chooses both analyst and supervisor, even though when it is a question of more than one supervisor some institutes will require that they be of both sexes. However, the candidate's choice of patient for the supervised cases will almost always be screened by the institute. It is a common procedure that prospective analysands are interviewed by a member of some kind of selection group elected by the institute before any contact between the candidate and his prospective analysand is allowed. Sometimes this screening procedure will take place with the supervising analyst conducting the interviews.

With the help of such procedures one hopes to supply the candidates with "suitable" analysands, and spare them from those with severe character disorders or those who might be presumed to terminate their analyses before any substantial analytic process has started to evolve. Such intentions, however, often turn out to be sweet expectations counteracted by a reality where it seems to be somewhat of an inevitability that the supervised cases turn out to be considerably more complicated than one would wish.

One additional intention behind the procedure to "supply" candidates with analysands is that the analytical relationship should be "clean." For their transferential matrix to develop undisturbed, both parties should be unknown to one another before the analysis.

The fundamental institutional functions of the supervised cases are the same as those of the training analyses. Supervision is an instrument for validating the selection of candidates. In conducting supervised cases the candidate learns how to do psychoanalysis. In this process lies a significant part of the normalization of the candidate: "the psychoanalytic techniques that are taught are also vehicles for teaching ideology" (Steltzer 1986:67).

The Pedagogic Conflict

One might think that with the abundance of literature that deals with various aspects of supervision within psychoanalytic training and also within general psychotherapeutic practice, the issue would be well covered. But that does not seem to be the case.

Wallerstein, for example, writes that "though the supervisory process has increasingly emerged over recent decades as the central vehicle in the teaching of psychoanalysis and psychoanalytic psychotherapy, there is still a much-decried paucity of literature on its nature and its vicissitudes" (1997:xiii). After decades of investigation and reflection concerning supervision within analytical training, considerable differences still prevail—not least in the United States—as to what supervision is, how it should be conducted, what the central problems are, or how the candidate should be evaluated.

Baudry writes that "in contrast to clinical work, which is informed by a complex systematized theory and technique, supervision is essentially still an uncharted territory" (1993:590). This very lack of a common ground contributes to the fact that "the personality of the analytic teacher plays a more significant role in supervision than in any other clinical teaching" (Fleming and Benedek 1964:73).[40] The general insecurity issuing from this "is compounded by an almost total absence of guidelines about supervision in our analytic institutes" (Baudry 1993:590).[41]

Weiss and Fleming, for example, reach the conclusion that little has been discussed concerning what might be expected from the supervisor's report or how the institute should make use of the information contained in it. They do, however, suggest the following categories: (1) sensitivity to unconscious meaning; (2) interpretive skill; (3) a capacity for self-analysis; (4) a capacity for grasping the analytic situation and process; (5) the ability to discuss cases in theoretical terms (1975:194). But, it is the same with this enumeration as with many others that the categories are self-evident and not followed up with a deeper discussion.

On the whole, there is a general lack of discussion of the true meanings and intentions of supervision, just as there seems to be no dialogue concerning negative effects of supervision (Szecsödy 1994:122). How are we to understand this obvious silence concerning the essence and function of supervision—or even its philosophy?

I would like to suggest that this lack of generally accepted conceptions of the meaning and goals of supervision has to do with a fundamental conflict within the supervisory situation as such—possibly not only when it is part of a training system, which is to say before any syncretistic dilemma or problem having to with the supervisor being a representative of the institution would show. What I have in mind is a *pedagogic conflict* that has to do with the supervisor having to be at one and the same time an educational authority *and* a mentor:

> Unlike a teacher, who most often is theoretically inclined and supports the learning of facts, and supervisors who may be either theoretically or practically oriented, mentorship is more personal and relies upon mutual exchange. Teachers and supervisors are usually aware of how things should be conducted, knowing the right answers, whereas the pupil is the one to benefit from their knowledge. . . . But, even if the mentor has an educative function, it is above all the problems and questions brought up by the pupil that are to be addressed. A well-functioning mentorship should promote the development of both parties. . . . Mentorship implies that two persons, a mentor and his pupil, have agreed upon reaching mutually accepted goals. The mentor should be a judicious person with a broad

and deep experience of life who, through his knowledge and experience, engagedly and with warmth of heart is willing to support a younger person's individual development and progress. [Lindgren 1997:281]

On the one hand, the supervisor is meant to be a guiding colleague; on the other, by dint of his greater experience, he is not only the one who is expected to know more, but also the one who will evaluate the candidate. As we saw in the quotation at the beginning of this chapter, Freud included psychoanalysis and education in that group of professions he deemed to be "impossible," which is to say that one could be sure to achieve unsatisfying results. The pedagogic conflict is presumably present in most educational projects. When it comes to the supervised cases, I would like to suggest that it is the pedagogic conflict that underlies the uncertainty—as to the goals, means, technique, and philosophy of supervision—that still prevails. This is such a problematic mixture of roles, so difficult to combine, that it remains hard to define what supervision is or what it should be.[42]

The pedagogic conflict exists, for example, in the state of tension in all psychoanalytical/psychotherapeutic supervision between what is usually called a "patient-oriented" versus a "therapist-oriented" perspective. Within the former, supervisor and supervisee focus their attention upon the analysand and the analytic process, especially the transferential process. Within the latter, the focus of supervision is on the supervisee's reactions, his blind spots, and countertransferences. The evident interest in the transference–countertransference interaction that has prevailed during the last twenty years or so has presumably reinforced the tendency toward therapist-oriented supervision.

The distinction between these two approaches to supervision has had a tendency to polarize, and the subject will most certainly remain an issue for discussion for a long time to come: "Whether supervision is primarily or exclusively an educational (didactic) experience or a therapeutic (emotionally corrective) one is not yet settled. . . . which kind of an experience should supervision be, didactic or therapeutic?" (Ornstein 1967:449). In practice, all good (undogmatic) supervision presumably would include a dialectical movement between the two perspectives (see Ekstein and Wallerstein 1958, Chapter 14; for a view on supervision from an intersubjective perspective, see Berman 2000).

If, however, the supervisor's function as mentor should derail and the therapist-oriented perspective become too one-sided, supervision runs the risk of becoming a form of therapy or analysis of the candidate. Then the supervision becomes a competitor to the candidate's analysis, an effect practically all commentators agree must not come to be (see below concerning the syncretism of supervision). Baudry, for example, writes that all attempts on the part of the supervisor at addressing the deeper personal motives behind the candidate's difficulties and conflicts in working with his patients are to be ruled out; all that may be brought within the supervisory situation itself are such elements that constitute direct interferences with the candidate's proper functioning in the clinical situation and in supervision (1993:594). Grinberg states it quite succinctly: "The candidate should be treated as a colleague and not as a patient" (1970:375).

As to the supervisor's function as teacher, Bibring writes that "the control-analyst must play the part of an elder brother: the candidates are not his pupils but his colleagues" (1937:371). Again, the mentor function, but this time as a counterweight to the disturbing effects of a supervision that tends to become too instructive: "pedagogical tendencies in supervision seem to me to be responsible for much of the persecutory climate that so often prevails in the psychoanalytical training in our institutes" (Haesler 1993:548).

The two views on supervision give rise to differing demands as to what the candidate should report to his supervisor concerning his work. One common model will expect the candidate to supply his supervisor with a precise written account of one or more of the last week's sessions. This may be handed over to the supervisor in advance or presented at their scheduled meeting. Such a model of reporting seems to be most congruent with the patient-oriented view of supervision, as the emphasis is placed upon the clinical material presented.

The competing model would invite the candidate to spontaneously bring up during the supervision session what occurs to him concerning his work with the analysand. This form of reporting emulates the free-association process of the clinical situation. For the candidate's associations to be meaningful, it seems natural that the supervisor would assume a more therapist-oriented stance, where the candidate's manner of speaking about the analysand—for example, his inconsistencies or one-sidedness in describing the analysand—would be the object of the supervisor's attempts at understanding and interpreting his transformations in relation to the analysand.

The Syncretism of Supervision

Hanns Sachs was invited to move from Vienna to Berlin with the specific mission to establish himself as the first training analyst. He soon found that it was difficult to combine the tasks of analyzing candidates, supervising them, and, in addition, discussing with them various theoretical topics. To evade the confusion of analytical and pedagogical aims, the Berlin Institute upheld a strict and deliberate barrier between the functions of training analyst and supervisor (Bernfeld 1962:464; see also Sachs 1947).

During the same period the opposite view that the analyst was the most suited supervisor did, however, occur, the rationale being that he would be privy to the candidate's unconscious conflicts like no one else. There were spokesmen for this view in Vienna, but above all in Budapest, where the Berlin model was regarded to be superficial: "In my view . . . the more correct procedure is for the control-analysis to be conducted throughout by the candidate's own training-analyst" (Kovács 1936:350–351).[43] It was thought that such a model would guarantee that the personal obstacles standing in the way of the candidate's professional development would be adequately treated, as the analyst had the opportunity to switch between his two functions and allow his knowledge of the candidate to alternately fecundate both areas.

Debell (1963) establishes that no thorough criticism or refutation of Kovács's standpoint exists in the literature. Seemingly—and without discussion—the principle of separating personal analysis from pedagogical aims was unanimously accepted by the end of the second epoch. For several decades, all training institutes have adhered to the principle that the training analyst and the supervisor should never be the same person for a particular candidate.

Even though things never came to be arranged the way the Budapest analysts wished them to be, there did arise a sort of field of tension between the two functions that would linger on as a variant of the syncretistic dilemma. During the forties and fifties proposals were made to the effect that training analysts and supervisors should engage in mutual discussions to consider the candidate (see, for example, Blitzsten and Fleming 1953). The almost total victory of the nonreporting system has made all such ideas outmoded. Nevertheless, it is still in our day a widespread requirement that the candidate be in analysis as long as he conducts at least the first of his supervised cases (see Bibring 1954:172), and in some institutes he is required to remain in analysis for the whole period of his training. The demand for psychoanalysis is usually justified by the above-mentioned conception that problems cropping up along the road may be brought up for treatment with the training analyst.

Thomä poses a reasonable question in this connection: "How often do candidates bring up in their own analysis what they have found disturbing in the therapies? What are the subjects that the candidate feels he cannot discuss with his supervision analyst?" (1993:36). To the second of Thomä's queries there is the common reply that supervision is not meant to be therapy or analysis. Instead, there is the more or less tacit agreement between all parties involved that the candidate turn to his training analyst to find help with the personal obstacles and problems that emerge during the course of his supervised work. Seldomly will the supervisor also be expected to encourage the candidate to bring certain issues from the supervised cases to be disentangled in the personal analysis. These may be things like the so-called blind spots, tenacious countertransference reactions that will not lend themselves to being transformed into meaningful interpretations but are instead acted out in relation to the analysand, reactions of defiance toward the institute or its representatives that are difficult to come to grips with, and so forth.

Here is a problem that connects with the first of Thomä's questions, but that I actually have not encountered in the literature. It has to do with the remarkable deviation from the otherwise prevailing view on analytical praxis taken for granted by those who promulgate such a relationship between supervision and training analysis. When given free rein, the psychoanalytic process, as we saw in Chapter 2, will develop according to the inner dynamics of the transference matrix. For something like that to take place, it is required that both parties' demands for quick solutions to pressing problems be set aside in favor of a more long-range process that in time might be expected to bring with it some kind of solution to even the more urgent issues.

A candidate who approaches his training analyst with problems issuing from his supervised cases with the hope of solving them so that he may continue his task in a more appropriate way actually brings in a request that goes against the grain of the very idea of psychoanalysis. It is, of course, up to the training analyst to decide how to reply to such a request and he surely has the possibility to interpret it as a defense against the power of the transference relationship or as an unrealistic perception of what the analytical process is capable of handling. But to the extent that candidate and analyst both share the understanding that the training analysis should serve such a goal, the analysis runs the risk of becoming a therapy when the process is allowed to be disturbed by urgent calls for help. Thus the syncretistic dilemma may creep into the training analysis because those involved have not sufficiently freed themselves from the idea that the personal analysis should be part of the overall pedagogic endeavor. So when a candidate overcomes the resistance against turning to his training analyst that Thomä seems to presuppose, the paradoxical outcome may be a training analysis that is not fully analytical. This will, among other things, leave the candidate with insufficient preparation for the task of facing his own analysands within the transference matrix, as was described above.

The institute's demand for (a training) analysis may also give rise to complications of a kind touched upon above. If, for example, some time before his training, an applicant has had a protracted and, in particular, a satisfying personal analysis based on a consciously felt need for help and with all the transference reactions and emotional turmoil belonging to a therapeutic analysis, he will in many instances be asked to submit himself to yet another one so that the requirement for a training analysis is met. A second analysis, then, to the candidate—and possibly also to the training analyst—will be felt to be unnecessarily imposed and a waste of time and money. Thus, as Pfeffer writes, during the period that he is under supervision, the candidate runs the risk of becoming a "captive patient" when he cannot terminate his analysis at his own discretion, a circumstance which, among other things, contributes to his becoming subservient to his training analyst (1974:80). This risk of becoming a subservient captive is one reason some discussants recommend that the personal analysis be terminated before the training begins: "It would appear to be in the best interests of both the student in training and the patient whose supervised analysis he undertakes that this ought not to be recommended until the student's analysis is in the stages of resolution or is satisfactorily ended" (Gitelson 1948:209).

Intimacy and Control

Another factor strongly influencing the supervised cases in psychoanalytic training is the fact that supervision is an intimate experience. In a way this is in the nature of things, but it becomes considerably reinforced as the reason for supervision taking place

at all is that the candidate is engaged in an ongoing analytic process that in itself is characterized by a high degree of intimacy.

> The supervisory process requires on the part of the supervisee
> a considerable amount of personal involvement and degree of
> revelation of the workings of his or her mind and sharing of
> emotions. This process creates intimacy and is also quite threat-
> ening. In contrast to the analytic relationship in which patients
> are assured of an impartial, nonjudgmental reception, super-
> visees know all the time that they will be judged and evalu-
> ated by their supervisor and that to a greater or lesser degree
> advancement in their careers is dependent on the type of evalu-
> ation they receive. [Baudry 1993:597]

Due to the fragility with which the candidate approaches the supervisor, supervision "has been considered almost as private and
confidential as analysis itself" (Fleming and Benedek 1964:73). But
the authors go on to say: "As long as this attitude persists very
little can be known about what happens in this teaching–learning
situation" (p. 73).

The institute's demand for control evidently collides with the
fragility of intimacy. Once the reporting system was abandoned
practically all over the world, we have been forced to bow before
the fact that the training analysis is (in principle) an inaccessible
territory of which nothing may be asked, and for that reason
evaluations are nowadays seldom made on the basis of open or
veiled communications coming from the training analyst. Therefore the supervised cases have come to be the most important
source of knowledge concerning the candidate's development
with respect to analytical competence and professional identity,
just as well as his personality (or character), his peculiarities, and
his unconscious psychic conflicts and problems. It is then part of
the supervisor's duty to report to the training institute: "The
supervisor, as a member of a training institute, has not only a
status, but also the power and responsibility to judge, evaluate
and influence the status of the candidate, the trainee" (Szecsödy
1994:129).

We can conclude that the relationship between intimacy and control constitutes a structural conflict encumbering the supervised cases, variously obstructing the candidate's work, and in the long run also leaving traces in his continued professional development. The decisive stumbling block is, of course, the fact that the candidate is inhibited by a feeling of being controlled:[44]

"The supervisee . . . is constantly being watched by his supervisor. Not having full grasp of the situation and the process, the recurrent, intrusive 'What am I supposed to do?' leads to a considerable loss of spontaneity" (Ornstein 1967:451). The candidate's feeling of insecurity easily makes the supervisor appear to be a strong authority: "I would say that my work was heavily burdened by my superego. My supervisors . . . became superego surrogates" (Thickstun 1985:187). One more or less automatic reply to this kind of problem so often tends to be the classical: "More analysis!" But even if neurotically colored attitudes toward authorities are mitigated through analysis, the fact remains that the candidate is constantly monitored by both his supervisor and the institute. The conflict between intimacy and control is a reality that is not undone, even by skillfully conducted training analyses.[45] For that very reason the supervisor and the institute must take into account that the candidate's truly creative clinical giftedness will in all probability come to the fore only once he has finished his training (see Meerlo 1952).

If control leads to the candidate's becoming inhibited and he is thereby hindered from doing and showing his best, a feeling of insecurity will permeate the whole supervisory project; it will be difficult for the supervisor to feel that he has a grip on what is taking place. It might not be so difficult to distinguish those candidates who are clearly untalented or harmful to their analysands (even if it can be quite troublesome for all parties involved to actually expel them).[46,47] What is considerably worse is that potentially good candidates are not given the opportunity to develop their full capacity when they lack the courage to step out and risk themselves in the encounter with the analysand.

The analytical setting—of which the candidate is trained to be the keeper—includes, as we saw above, the implicit promise that all that is said and done within the walls of the analyst's office is subjected to the strictest confidentiality. It is then quite apparent that supervision is a direct violation of the fundamental ethic underlying the analytical encounter. As with clinical presentations or the publishing of material from the analytical process (with or or without the analysand's consent), supervision is a betrayal of the subjective dimension of psychoanalytical treatment, its warmth and intimacy.

Therefore supervision will leave a trace of culpability and a bit of confusion in the supervisee (cf. Britton 1997:11–12), not least because he finds it difficult to gauge the extent of his treason; not only is the supervisor the recipient of his information, but in a much more indirect fashion so is the institute. And so we may also find that the candidate's attempts to exculpate himself by, for example, being vague in his presentation of the process, will contribute to the supervisor's impression that what is going on is less clear than it need be.

And, to the general feeling of a lack of clarity as to what is being conveyed to the supervisor from the candidate's analytical work is added the fundamental fact that we can never really know what takes place in the encounters between our colleagues and their analysands: "This is one reason why clinical presentations are often such charged, emotional occasions. They offer the hope of communicating to our colleagues what we cannot show them, of putting a professionally sanctioned breach in our rule of confidentiality, of overcoming the isolation and loneliness to which we are condemned by the need for privacy in our profession" (Spurling 1997:65). To communicate that which cannot be shown: the problem would seem evident in the relationship between the professional psychoanalyst and the layman, but is actually just as urgent in the communication between colleagues and therefore also in supervision. Analytical confidentiality excludes the presence of a third person, and therefore the supervisor will always have only secondhand material at his disposal—whether the candidate offers him a spontaneous oral presentation of the sessions or tries to write down the best reconstruction of the dialogue that he is capable of, yes, even if he were to present taped recordings of the sessions.

The gist of this is that the supervisor can never feel truly certain of whether or not the candidate to some extent is deceiving him—be it that he is deceiving him only because he is deceiving himself, or to protect the analysand, or to defend his own personal vulnerability.[48] The attempt to communicate around the experience that supervision claims to have as its object will always suffer from serious shortcomings. Therefore the supervisor's own experience is so important: where communication is lacking he must fill in with his own knowing. In spite of this, however, a structurally conditioned propensity for suspicion tends to be inherent in supervision, which therefore will continue to cause it to be perceived as a deficient instrument for evaluation (at least when compared with the training analysis).

To illustrate how this suspicion works and what consequences it may have, I take the liberty to digress and refer to an investigation carried out at an anonymous training facility called "Eastern Institute" (Dulchin and Segal 1982a). At the time, most American institutes still relied upon the classical reporting system described above. However, at the Eastern, it was decided to preserve the integrity of the personal analysis as far as possible and therefore the Institute implemented a nonreporting system that distinguished between analytical work and evaluation. To be sure, the training analysts did have the double function of both analysts and supervisors, but never in relation to the same candidate.

It turned out, though, that under certain specific circumstances Eastern Institute was incapable of maintaining the principle of nonreporting, despite the fact, it might be added, that its members appeared to have felt rather proud over having adopted the new system. For example, Dulchin and Segal describe how a training analyst managed to influence the selection committee in such a way that a certain person was not chosen for training. His way of conveying his message was to tell one of the members of the committee, in seclusion, that the applicant was unsuitable. Without in any way having to—or, considering the "illegitimate" way in which he had acquired his information, without being able to—substantiate his claims, the recipient of this information later said at a committee conference: "Be very careful and watchful when you interview this guy. I hear he is a psychopath" (Dulchin and Segal 1982a:17). Those who then interviewed the person in question could, of course, guess that it was the applicant's analyst who had submitted the information, and on that basis they estimated the judgment as valid.

The authors also describe how similar actions could be employed to influence the evaluation of candidates already in training. In instances where the candidate's analysts were themselves members of the committees where their analysands were discussed, it would be enough that they simply grunt or make a conspicuous gesture to indicate their dislike of the direction the discussion was taking.

Dulchin and Segal go on to deal with the various forces underlying such flagrant violations against a self-imposed rule of nonreporting and nonintervention. The first and—in the view of many—most "forgivable" of these forces is the intent to guard the safety of future analysands. The authors do underscore, however, that considerations of that kind could not be wholly separated from the interest in safeguarding the goodwill of the Institute. Similarly, it would have negative repercussions on a training analyst's reputation should his name be associated with an analyst who was inferior or even destructive to those he had in treatment. "The violations of confidentiality, therefore, expressed ultimately the need of all analysts to maintain their standing, as individuals and as members of a particular institute, in the psychoanalytic world" (Dulchin and Segal 1982a:19).

To be sure, there are institutes where one does follow the rule that the (training) analyst in question always be requested to leave the room while his candidate is up for discussion; that may even be the prevailing procedure today. Such a system would certainly reduce the possibilities of intervening directly in the discussions, but would not obliterate all available channels for such influence. Apart from the forces and interests just mentioned, there are additional reasons for a committee to remain sensitive to what signals may be coming from a training analyst. Dulchin and Segal write that the supervisors at Eastern Institute were easily influenced by signals coming from the training analyst for the simple reason that they themselves felt that they lacked real insight into the candidates' work. They had to rely upon secondhand information in the form of candidate reports from the consulting room, but never had any firsthand observations of candidates in the clinical situation. Because they were themselves analysts to other candidates, they knew that the knowledge they had from the supervisions they conducted was shallower than that from analyses. Thus they would hesitate to reach a decision on the sole basis of information coming from the supervision and allowed themselves to be influenced by third-party information coming from the analytical situation.

The authors point out that despite the described routines for breach of confidentiality being applied with apparent ease ("Senior analysts . . . tended to see nothing problematic in the use of such information" [Dulchin and Segal 1982b:34]),[49,50] they would be used only in such cases when serious problems had cropped up. Likewise, one could conclude that confidentiality was always respected when the supervisors shared the same high regard of the candidate with the analyst. One of the really serious aspects of a system of information such as this is that presumably, as the information shared is always disclosed in separate chambers or by insinuation, it is extremely difficult to evaluate or question it. The authors conclude with a disconcerting perspective: "The incompatibility between psychoanalysis (with its requirements of candor and confidentiality) and the training of psychoanalysts in organizations (with their requirements of careful evaluation) is always likely to entail the institutional use of third parties' analytic confidences" (1982b:37).

Rustin writes: "It is a remarkable achievement of this community that it succeeds in containing and controlling all this out-of-place information in such a way that it can be used in necessary ways, without destroying the confidence and limits on which analysis depends" (1985:149). It is not only remarkable but admirable how analysts, with such precision for the most part, are able to manage all the very delicate information that has been left in their custody, but when it comes to their training system there is apparently a communicative subgrowth that threatens good confidentiality (we will return to this problem in the next chapter).

Some authors wish to handle the difficulties connected with supervision by lessening its importance: "Supervision is overemphasized, bureaucratic, and too much patient-care-oriented. It prolongs a dependent student status, creates multiple identifications, and delays finding an independent, personal style" (Bak 1970:19).

Robert Langs advocates a supervision model based on the setting of the analytic situation and suggests a nonreporting system for supervision:

> The best solution available at the moment appears to be allowing supervisees to select a supervisor from a roster of certified supervisors, and for the supervision to be conducted on a private basis without reports on the supervisee to any outside party. The supervisee's graduation from or certification by the training programme would then depend upon case presentations to a committee of the institute from which the supervisee's therapist and supervisor are excluded. [1997:132]

The Supervisor's Function as Mentor

The transmission of knowledge through individual supervision of the kind practiced in psychoanalytic training has a certain likeness to the kind of apprenticeship that has been common in preindustrial societies. For economic reasons apprenticeship has become scarce in modern forms of education, but as supervision it has had somewhat of a renaissance and seems to be increasingly common at the end of different professional training programs. Such professional supervision

> presupposes that the supervisor and the supervisee share the same practice. Supervision then deals with a current and tangible work situation. The content of supervision must be re-

lated to professional competence and professional functions.
The supervisor's primary task is to lay the ground for the supervisee to develop his professional role by establishing an
identity and expanding his competence for the work at hand.
[Selander and Selander 1989]

Despite all obscurities and difficulties connected with the
supervised cases, the fact seems to remain that the deep-going
dialogue that characterizes analytical supervision is an exceptionally privileged pedagogic model. The high ratio between supervision sessions and encounters with the analysand (usually 1:4 or
1:5), in combination with the duration of the contact, distinguishes
psychoanalytic supervision from that of other professional training programs in that it offers a unique provision of individually
adapted support for the development of a professional identity.
And despite the very tangible difficulties encumbering the system, the supervised cases seem to comprise that experience within
analytic training in which candidates tend to feel that they receive
considerable help and support and learn something very substantial (see Baudry 1993:590). Supervision is often a satisfying experience for the supervisor also, who—unlike in the analyses he
conducts—is here provided with a "longed for social contact and
free dialogue" (Grinberg 1970:376).

How, then, to formulate the goals of such an activity? Apart
from the aim mentioned above, the essence of which is to gauge
the effects of the candidate's training analysis via the moment of
supervision, Bibring also mentions that the task of the control
analyst is "(1) to make sure how far the candidate grasps . . . the
structure of the neurosis with which he is dealing, the various
phases of the analytic situation, both as a whole and in detail, and
the course which the analysis is taking; (2) to keep a check on his
technique and especially on his interpretations" (1937:370).

The whole thing became a bit more formalized when the APA,
in the middle of the fifties, specified its "Minimal standards for
the training of physicians in psychoanalysis." This prescription,
which is just as representative as any other, describes the aim and

function of supervised cases as: (1) instructing the candidate in the management of the psychoanalytic method; (2) helping him to attain therapeutic skillfulness based on the understanding of analytic material; (3) observing his work and deciding whether his personal analysis has been successful; (4) judging his level of maturity and stability over a protracted period of time (APA 1956:718).

As mentioned, a list of goals or virtues will easily be misleading—not least because it is most often construed to meet the needs of the institute. As an alternative method for describing the meaning of a certain aspect of training, one could, for example, describe the stages of supervision that a candidate is expected to pass. Ornstein suggests four such stages: (1) The candidate must learn how it "feels" to be an analyst and be present in this very intimate situation with another human being where he is receiving so much trust; (2) he must learn to act and express himself like a psychoanalyst; (3) he must learn how an analyst thinks; (4) he must learn to listen with evenly suspended attention (1967:451–459).

Instead of repeating the always equally unsatisfying attempts at making lists of desired characteristics, abilities, or signs of maturity, following Ornstein I would suggest rather that one concentrate on what central issues confront the candidate during the supervisory process. I do not intend to cover this area now, for that would require a separate investigation. I merely wish to emphasize the importance of the candidate's finding a path along which he will personally discover the matrix of transference as an affectively shared reality. This presupposes that he has had the opportunity to experience in his personal analysis the mental space of transference as the central playground of the analytic encounter with an atmosphere all its own.

A recurrent difficulty in all supervision seems to be the transmission of precisely this experience of transference, so that the candidate and the analysand together may grasp it as a living presence, feeling secure enough to safeguard their freedom and motility within its bounds. One important reason for this difficulty seems to me to be what was mentioned above, namely that training analyses display a tendency to remain "cool." If the candidate in supervision has had only a diffuse experience of transference, he will encounter difficulties in finding and identifying the transferential dimension in his own work. There is a definite risk that this problem will remain a structural weakness in the analytical training system as long as the candidate subjects himself to analytic treatment due more to pedagogical requirements than out of personal need.

However, when the candidate has managed to accommodate himself to the matrix of transference that he shares with his analysand it is most important that the supervisor assist him with all available means in mustering the courage to remain there and conduct his actions in a warm and genuinely personal manner. To be a fellow human being of utmost importance for his analysand is a demanding task that takes a long time to master. For this to happen, the supervisor's grasp of the candidate's strengths and weaknesses is indispensable so that the latter will have enough self-confidence in his ability to handle the crisis that inevitably will come when one day he is to conduct psychoanalytic work on his own (more of this in the following chapter). In this, the function of the supervisor resembles mentorship more than anything else.[51]

Just as we could see above in connection with the training analysis, it is a widespread notion that identification plays an important part in the transmission of the sought-after abilities: "The most effective influence, pedagogically, in the supervisory situation probably is the identification with the supervisor" (Arlow 1963:590; see also, for example, Szecsödy 1994:121). But, because the concept lacks a clearly elaborated definition and is used to designate a number of differing phenomena it remains problematic. And, to be honest, what in the supervisory situation would the candidate identify with (emulate)? He does not meet the supervisor in his function of analyst, and the supervisory situation is certainly not an opportunity for the supervisor to tell of his own cases and experiences. And it is surely not the art of supervising that is to be identified with.

As in my previous discussion concerning identification with the training analyst, I would rather wish to stress *the internalization of the supervisor's function*. Haesler writes that "the outcome of the supervisory process will eventually be an internalisation of the supervisor's functioning, and this inner functioning of the internalised supervisor will be crucial for the competent functioning of the candidate as future psychoanalyst" (1993:555). In line with my previous formulation concerning internalization as the absorption of intersubjective relationships and their transformation into subjective structures, I would suggest that we understand internalization in the supervisory experience as the acquisition of a disposition to execute the same functions that the candidate met with in his supervisor.

Which, then, are the functions to be internalized? It lies beyond the scope of this book to establish an exhaustive list of the functions that can be internalized in the supervisory situation, but there are two that seem to me to be exceedingly important and in fact not often recognized as such. The first of these touches upon what I discussed above concerning the training analysis: one of the primary positive functions of psychoanalytic training is to make of the candidate a keeper of the analytical setting. Calef and Weinshel suggest that it is the analyst's task to be the "conscience of the analysis": he is "the 'keeper of the analytic process' who has the responsibility of maintaining the psychoanalytic work and process" (1980:279).[52]

To be the keeper of the analytical setting is a demanding ethical goal that permeates all psychoanalytic training. There is most probably nothing comparable to substantiate the ethos of psychoanalysis as the analyst's way of safeguarding the setting so that the best possible preconditions will prevail for good psychoanalytic work to develop. Without its specific setting, psychoanalytic work would rapidly deteriorate. There is all reason to expect, therefore, that the supervisor's function as the conscience of the analysis be gradually internalized by the candidate so that he, in time, may himself be the keeper of the analytic setting.

We find here, however, a difference in relation to the kind of internalization mentioned above in connection with the training analysis. The internalization of the training analyst's function is the direct result of *being engaged in interaction* with him. In the supervisory situation things tend to look a bit different because the candidate, as we noted, does not interact with the supervisor as analyst. The essential communication will rather show in the supervisor's ways of guiding the candidate in daring to affectively reach out and touch the analysand, to be important, or to keep alive a sense of warmth and caring.

Regarding a sense of warmth and caring, the most frequent term seems to be "empathy"—or *Einfühlung*, as Freud wrote. The English "empathy" is an invention by Strachey from Greek roots. In its Greek-as-it-were-English garb, I have always felt disinclined to embrace this term with any enthusiasm because it sounds like an identificatory feeling insight of a kind that must be based upon an objectivation of the analysand, where "I can understand you because I can very well imagine what kind of situation you are in." But, analytical work *within the transference*—that is to say where both parties are submerged in the matrix of transference and make themselves responsible to this fact—does not depend upon the analyst trying to "embrace" his analysand with a vicarious work of mentation. Working within the transference creates an immediate and affectively warm presence, not so that the analyst "shows his feelings," as one tends to say when things are allowed to spill a bit, but through his allowing his affects to be the foundation for what he has to say. Precisely because this is so difficult, one of the supervisor's most important tasks is to aid the candidate in (re)finding a composed attitude of caring.

THE THEORETICAL SEMINARS

The aims of education run contrary to those of psychoanalysis. Education implies fixity of meaning and the illusion of mastery associated with understanding. The power of description, theoretical formulation, models, causal links, facts, stories,

myths, fictions—whatever constitutes the explanatory substance of educational discourses—derives from points of fixity, from gaps being filled with fixed meanings. Education
always aims to fill a gap and is fundamentally predicated upon
the assumption that all gaps are fillable, while psychoanalysis
aims to help you live with the inevitable gap at the middle of
your existence. The built-in dynamic of the analysand's desire
subverts the educational project while the requirement for closure in educational discourse forecloses desire. Thus they are
antithetical. [Hall 1996:70]

The arrangement of the theoretical seminars will vary, depending on which institute one is studying. Generally, though, they take
place during the course of three to five years, and then usually in
the form of evening classes one or two days a week. Usually major
courses will be given to cover the following areas: (1) general psychoanalytic theory; traditionally, Freud's writings—case histories
and theoretical texts—play a central role here; (2) clinical theory,
embracing general and specific psychopathology, theories of neurosis and psychosis, and diagnostics; (3) technical seminars to guide
the candidates' supervised work. There may also be courses dealing with subjects such as the history of psychoanalysis or epistemology and the philosophy of science. Besides these theoretical
courses there are the important case seminars where a candidate will
usually present to a group some ongoing work under supervision
from a training analyst (less often it will be an older and experienced [training] analyst making such a presentation). In some societies there will be special requirements such as the writing and
presentation of a paper, either to become a member at all or to attain what in some societies is called "full membership."

Perhaps to a greater extent than when it comes to the supervised cases, the theoretical seminars belong to that part of psychoanalytic training that is the least investigated. Dorn writes that
the analytic training institution is a "teacher-centered rather than
student-centered organization" (1969:249), a circumstance that
manifests itself in various ways in the form and content of the
theoretical seminars.

Thus, for example, one almost always structures seminars as if one were teaching children, with a fixed curriculum and a specified quantum of knowledge to be acquired. Seldomly does one take after the model of the university and let the candidates compile their own theoretical seminar by choosing from a menu of available courses. We are far from the ideal held forth by Anna Freud when in 1966 she spoke of a future psychoanalytic institute where "theoretical courses will be no more than a method of guiding the candidate toward independent reading" (1971:234). In the name of uniformity and predictability all candidates are to be cast in the same mold, a way of arranging things that will not leave much room for independent thought. To be sure, the interest in research and the promotion of theoretical work are practically totally forgotten in psychoanalytic training. Schachter and Luborsky report that at the time of writing (1998) only four of twenty-two institutes in the United States have courses in analytical research in their programs.

The prevailing offering of courses is often criticized for being shaped by outmoded ideals: "When psychoanalytic institutes were first formed . . . Freud's contributions were approached in an uncritical way" (Arlow and Brenner 1988:6). As a result of this, the authors continue, it is all too common to see how a multitude of training institutes put too much emphasis on antiquated texts and issues. "We are one of the few scientific disciplines that uses as primary texts books that are 75 to 80 years old" (Arlow 1982:13–14). It is, of course, important that candidates be imparted an understanding of the history of the discipline, but "Freud's writings are most often disseminated as if they were holy texts" (Cremerius 1987:1069). For example, it is widely known that Freud's clinical cases—say, "Dora" or "The Rat Man"—to our day are still promulgated as exemplary for candidates in training (see also Kernberg 1986:810):

Consider for a moment the situation of the candidate who approaches his first supervised case. In favorable situations, this may happen any time from the last trimester of the first year to the middle of the second year of courses. What preparations

does he bring with him to this fresh challenge? [Here Arlow
enumerates some early texts by Freud.] Considering the selection of the texts . . . and the order in which they are offered,
we have to conclude that, as a process, this kind of psychoanalytic curriculum encourages imitation of the master rather
than independent and critical examination of the data. [Arlow
1982:14–15]

In a report from a congress on psychoanalytic training, Calef poses
a question that perhaps epitomizes the dilemma of psychoanalytic
education. He asks "whether the philosophical and educational
goals of the institutes are really the basis upon which the educational methods are designed, whether they represent a fit, and
really serve, psychoanalytic education" (1972:37). To give a ten-
tative answer to Calef's query, I would say that the analytic training system never really has thought—or has been able to think
through—its philosophical and pedagogic goals. To this whole
issue belongs the fact that the unknown quantity of analytic training—and thus also of the analytic instititution—is the analyst
himself. The documentation in this chapter has demonstrated that
we do not know what it is that constitutes a good analyst, or what
is required of a good candidate. Thus we cannot know fully what
it is that constitutes a good training system. It should come as no
surprise, then, that the methods of instruction are ill adapted to
the task when its nature remains so ill defined.

The lack of a philosophy for analytical training and perhaps
in particular for the acquisition of knowledge, has to do with a
conflict between the professional-clinical and the intellectual-
scientific interests, respectively. A profession, writes Bird, is
above all established to meet the demands and needs of the general public making it "essentially an applied field, dedicated first
and foremost to the application of knowledge, not to the extension of knowledge" (1968:516)—and therefore the "performance
of scientific work . . . is conspicuous by its absence among the
long list of requirements for membership in the analytic community" (Szasz 1958:601). Professionals are not attracted to seeing themselves as scientists, but are at the same time dependent

upon an existing, trustworthy, and solid body of knowledge to base their practices on.

Psychoanalytic training is clearly professionally clinically oriented—and so it should be. But although the professional-clinical interest is dependent upon an existing body of knowledge, surprisingly few tangible structures are erected to widen, deepen, and critically assess this body. Knowledge should somehow just be there. Preferably it should also function just like one self-deceptively likes to think it does: like a sturdy guide to the experience pertaining to the clinical situation (see the discussion in Chapter 2 on the use of theory). But substantive opportunities for theoretical work are seldom created.

It seems inevitable that sooner or later psychoanalysis will have to subject its own relationship to its knowledge and its theories to a radical evaluation, but to this day it still seems to be afflicted with a conspicuous ambivalence in that respect. On the one hand, one needs knowledge, while on the other it is treated not without a certain measure of contempt. A flagrant expression of the obviously ambivalent attitude of institutes in relation to the transmission of knowledge they are entrusted to guarantee comes to the fore in how scarce are formal methods of examination for the theoretical seminars (see Arlow 1982:7). "How often have we heard," asks Wallerstein (1972:600), "that someone has actually failed a course or been made to repeat it?"

5

THE SUPEREGO COMPLEX

Some years ago, in the context of a discussion with [Lore Schacht] about ways to increase the creativity of candidates in psychoanalytic training, [she] told me, with a smile: "Our problem is not so much to foster creativity but to try not to inhibit the creativity naturally stimulated by the nature of our work.

—O. Kernberg 1996:1031

Psychoanalysis is an activity that is practiced in the secluded and exclusive encounter between analyst and analysand. The rules of the setting require that no third party be allowed, and the norms and values that are presumed to guide all good and ethically sound work are cultivated within groups and communities that are separate from the practice itself: the training institutes and the societies.

As I attempted to describe in Chapter 2, the good of psychoanalysis resides in the very *praxis* of psychoanalysis, and when it proceeds in accordance with its intended ways analytic work is characterized by an aspiration that very well might be labeled "loving."[1] One would think that something similar could be expected of life within the psychoanalytic organizations. But things do not always match such expectations: there is often a clear distance between the immanent goods of the practice—its intended ways—and the organizational and institutional functions meant (among other things) to safeguard these goods. Briefly put, collegial relations between psychoanalysts are often characterized by obvious destructiveness.

The underlying problem might have to do with whether psychoanalysis can live with its institutions at all—or at least that we as yet have failed to invent that really good form that would harmoniously combine these two efforts. But this is surely not a phenomenon limited to psychoanalytical institutions. Precisely because of the way organizations and larger groups tend to function, manifestly destructive tendencies can root themselves and be transmitted from one generation to the next. Finding the good organizational and institutional form meets with considerable difficulty.

In the present investigation the emphasis is definitely on the dark aspects and their deforming effects. But to reasonably delve deeper into this, something must be said concerning the lasting ties with which the psychoanalyst is attached to the organizations he has created for himself. Without such a perspective the analyst would seem to be prepared to almost masochistically subject himself to his institutions, rather than reform or even depart from them when they threaten the very kernel of his praxis: "[W]hile many psychoanalysts are dissatisfied with the system of training, there is little enthusiasm for reform" (Thomä 1993:5).

To grasp the analyst's loyalty to his institutions we must take into account some fundamental circumstances surrounding his practice. First, psychoanalysis has always perceived itself to be alone in enemy territory, or at least seldom in the company of really close friends. In part, the alienation is self-inflicted in that psychoanalysts willingly cultivate the notion that no one but they really understands, that the insights of the discipline are quite sufficient, and that one needs no additional knowledge. Apparent negative consequences evolving from this attitude have been sectarianism, contempt for the surrounding world and its realities, and a well-groomed paranoia: "It is as if we do live with the illusion of always moving in a goldfish bowl with the world always breathlessly watching to see what our (omniscient) stand will be" (Wallerstein 1981a:296).

However true that picture may have been, it is equally important to remember that psychoanalysis really has had no good reasons for feeling at home in this world.[2] For reasons too many and too complicated to be detailed here, it is true that analysis has existed in a more or less manifest position of the outsider. And this despite, for example, its flourishing alliance with American psychiatry during the forties and the fifties, or the fact that it so often has shouldered the role of pet discipline to certain culturally fashionable groups and trends. Or despite psychoanalysis both in Europe and the United States having enjoyed support both from government-run and private insurance systems (although there are strong indications that all this is about to change radically, if it actually hasn't already—see the next chapter).

For, as things so often have shown themselves to be, allies may suddenly and without warning transform into indifferent onlookers or even vicious slanderers. On a collective level psychoanalysis has therefore striven to guarantee its own survival by defending strict demands for competence and quality. In this way, a striving for professional respectability has arisen, manifesting itself in strong organizations and a well-controlled training system where, for better or worse, a superego is cultivated and maintained that may well be designated as "orthodox," the function of which is to secure the survival of psychoanalysis as a stable discipline, together with a form of treatment that will be recognizable among different geographic locations and also over time. But, from just this complex array of causes issue the very problems that this investigation seeks to describe: "[O]ne may wonder how much this lack of external recognition as a discipline increases our need for rites, for secrecy, 'in' and 'out' groups, a secret language" (Orgel 1978:513; see also Rustin 1985).

When it comes to the clinically active psychoanalyst there are some specific conditions to be aware of, besides these social circumstances. Psychoanalytic work is a solitary enterprise that can be especially cumbersome. There are a multitude of obstacles to sharing with others the problems encountered, or to displaying to the world a good performance and thus receiving its appreciation—

a possibility available to most other professionals (should anyone want to listen). It is, of course, possible to make oneself known and to some extent even famous by publishing theoretical work or research—and such forms of reward are surely not to be underestimated—and within the smaller group of colleagues there is the possibility of advancing to the status of training analyst. But for the core activity itself, the principle of confidentiality puts a stop to practically all possibilities of finding appreciation for the work one carries out (except, perhaps, from the analysands themselves, whose affection and loyalty to some extent are always relative because they are in a position of dependency).

> The practice of psycho-analysis is a lonely business. There is probably no endeavour which makes greater demands on the capacity to be alone. Drastic reduction in consensual communication is conductive to regression beyond what is technically useful in the service of the analyzing ego. Infantile sources of stimulus-hunger are revived; the need for "narcissistic supplies" is aroused; the compensatory wish for participation in, and active control of, the external world is intensified. The analyst's immersion in the unconscious produces a kind of agoraphobic separateness which makes it important for him to find somewhere some fenced in common ground with others. Add to this the guilts and disappointments which attach to the difficulties of the therapeutic task, and it would be surprising indeed if there were no disillusionment, no need for validation in the eyes of others, no hankering after conventional scientific fraternity, no wish to be safely bound by ordinary rules and methods. [Gitelson 1963:526][3]

Professional self-reliance takes a long time to develop, and the analytic attitude is constantly exposed to eroding influences (see the section "Decisive Years," below). In the previous chapter the setting was presented as a prerequisite for the ethical trustworthiness of the psychoanalytic process, without which both clinical and theoretical work run the risk of foundering. Besides clinic and theory the analytic attitude stands as the third foundation of the analytic experience: let us say that the analytic attitude constitutes the subjective substratum in the analyst's person that is required for maintaining the setting.

There is tangible pressure weighing on psychoanalysis aimed at the analytic attitude and deriving partly from the deep wishes of analysands that we give them love rather than analyze them, and partly from the surrounding society, which finds it difficult to understand why one should allow single individuals to spend so much money and resources on an activity that cannot be unambiguously accounted for in terms of costs and benefits. The pressure inherent in expectations of this kind constitute a threat to the integrity of the psychoanalytic endeavor, and the analyst is forced to struggle to maintain the attitude of his profession in defiance of demands that it might be something different: a more open, accessible, cheaper, and quicker form of treatment—and in addition, more intelligible and less exclusive.

But to the threats to the analytic attitude also belong those forces that arise in the consulting room: "The analyst is continually drawn to do more than analyze, and his very humanness makes it difficult for him to invariably resist all the temptation" (Silverman 1985:177). This would apply in particular to the young analyst, who, for example, "may feel in danger of losing his patient to a therapist offering more direct gratification" (Dorn 1969:249).

> There is no analyst, subject to the daily spectrum of transference displacements, who does not know and feel the range of pressures to which this is put, from sexual to material to narcissistic. Basic trust is rightly tested and has to be earned. The capacity to use rather than to abuse transference cannot be taken for granted. Nor once achieved does it automatically continue for life. It needs to be worked at and constantly reaffirmed. [Rangell 1974:11; see also Schafer 1983]

The encounter with distress, helplessness, implacability, and irreparable loss and deficiency, together with strong expressions of despair and anxiety, expose the analyst to yet other forces that threaten to corrupt his attitude. To summarize, one could speak of the issues discussed here as a concern regarding the psycho-analyst's mental health.[4]

To remain stable in the face of the demands, threats, and dif-ficulties that the practice of the profession meets with, the ana-lytic community—institutionalized through societies and their constituent activities: training, congresses, colloquia, and super-visory contexts—sustains a psychoanalytic identity and a super-ego whose function for better or worse is to safeguard and transmit the ethos that alone will uphold that orientation which will allow psychoanalysis to be and remain what it is. To put it simply, you could say that psychoanalysts keep an eye on one another: "Vigilance is a part of the analyst's habit of mind, and in this task he is considerably aided by a social institution which keeps before him a useful mirror reflecting both himself and the contemporary world of similar experience, viz. the dis-cussions in the meetings of his psychoanalytical society" (Rickman 1951:219).

To evade the isolation brought on by the nature of the task, for the preservation of the analytic attitude, and to ensure the integrity of the analyst, collegial fellowship plays a very impor-tant role: "Scientific communications in a psychoanalytic society have not only the purpose of training and informing, but also reassure the group and each member individually about his psy-choanalytic identity" (Widlöcher 1983:38). Without his societies, institutes, and associations, the analyst easily feels stripped and exposed to a world where he is not at home: "When the fact of belonging to the institution is questioned, this may carry with it experiences of marginality, chaos or the end of the world" (Bernardi and Nieto 1992:143–144).

Thus arises a fear of altering existing structures, as if thereby all security were to be lost. Or even worse: to lose them through reform or decline—not to mention the threat of no longer being allowed to belong: "So many analysts are so very strongly identi-fied with the notion of *being* a psychoanalyst that, as far as they're concerned, maintaining that identity means belonging to a soci-ety" (Coltart, in Molino 1997:171). And all the while there resides in the analyst's confidence in his institutions the obvious paradox that the very same community is also marked by so much discord.

CONCEPTS AND THEIR USE

I wish to underscore that what is presented in this chapter is the depiction of *a* general structure and in no way a description of any single psychoanalytic society or other existing organization. It is my contention, however, that the intended general structure does prevail to a more or less prominent degree in most—not to say all—psychoanalytic organizations (and in all probability in organizational connections other than the purely psychoanalytic ones).

In Chapter 1 I introduced the term "the superego complex," which will here be used as a heuristic conceptual tool for opening up and studying the general structure. The complex itself comprises two substructures: "the professional superego" and "the institutional superego system." I regard the first one as an intrapsychic and private phenomenon, and the other as a system existing on a group level within psychoanalytic organizations. Superego and superego system mutually reinforce one another, and the complex thus constituted has the double function of being both prescriptive and proscriptive. In this double capacity the complex has great influence on the analyst's freedom and creativity, both in his praxis and in his theoretical work (later in this chapter I will supply more exhaustive definitions). It is the proscriptive aspect that will mainly be of interest to us in this investigation.

The reader will notice that in what follows I will cultivate a seemingly ahistorical form of presentation, where quotes from the forties and the nineties are mixed at will, as if we were dealing with one and the same decade. Shuffling decades in this fashion is a way of writing about conditions I consider to be typical—although not static—of a period extending over some sixty years, and is also a way of illustrating how well developed the self-understanding of the psychoanalytic institution has been during all this time.

It is in the nature of complexes that they do not easily lend themselves to simple definitions. To capture the complexity of our complex we will have to proceed as we did in the previous chapter: by investigating the small details, and especially those among which the roots of the complex may be expected to thrive. With alternating movements between descriptions and heuristic categorizations I hope to reach a point where it will in the end be possible to discern a totality. That totality can be grasped only if we begin by accepting the splits, gaps, and separations on which it rests. There is an obvious distance between the intrinsic values of psychoanalytical practice and the manner of functioning so often characteristic of psychoanalytic institutions. I would say that this is basically a question of a conflict between love and hate.

A STATE WITHIN THE STATE

The presence of a particular caste within psychoanalytic organizations (i.e., the group of training analysts) seems to provide an essential institutional hotbed for the general structure of the superego complex. This is not only a question of classes within the body of psychoanalysts, but also a very efficacious dynamic between the training analyst as an informal institution and the formal organization—in the way that the latter is delimited by a set of bylaws, whereas the former is not—which has been created to meet the needs and continued growth of psychoanalysis.

The institution of the training analyst is formed by a carefully selected circle that allows entry only to those with the highest qualifications. The pronounced requirement for absolute excellence, which at an early stage came to enclose this separate cadre among analysts, is directly connected with the striving for professionalism. It was understood that the respectability of both the treatment itself and the body of analysts would be dependent upon how well it could be made plausible to the general public that the psychoanalyst himself was well-analyzed: "In organizing our training, we should first of all look for competent training-analysts" (Lampl-de Groot 1954:187).

An Institution, Not an Organization

A profession which necessitates such an extensive and deep-going experience as the training analysis becomes, as a result, an organization in which emotional interpersonal relations are more significant than in any other profession.

—T. Benedek 1954:12

In some societies the training analyst is appointed at the institute's initiative; in others the analyst himself submits an application and will then have to undergo an evaluation procedure. For this task most societies or institutes have appointed a special group or committee. In particular, the larger societies have an evolved system of subgroups and committees, which also means—and this is important to keep in mind—that the training institute at large is not necessarily congruent with the body of training analysts.

The usual basic requirement for a training analyst is that during a number of years after matriculation—most often not less than five—he has been clinically active with psychoanalytic treatments at least half the time and that during that period he has conducted some four or five thousand sessions. In addition, he must be known to be a skilled clinician with a spotless reputation. In many societies it is required that the applicant present his work, either in writing or at a seminar or a clinical discussion. In some places it is also required that he publish some kind of theoretical work.[5] (And still, despite the demands, the fact remains that training analysts de facto constitute a group of colleagues with which the average analyst will be the least acquainted when it comes to their clinical abilities, as they most often do not present any case material [Cremerius 1987:1078; Kernberg 1986:799–800]).

Traditionally, the appointment to be a training analyst has meant that the person in question is authorized to conduct both analyses and supervision with candidates (A.-M. Sandler 1982:395). Today however, it is discussed in many quarters whether the training analyst shouldn't undergo some special training at the institute before he can supervise, as is already the rule at the Swedish Psychoanalytic Society.[6]

> The career of the average training analyst, qua training analyst, is a relatively brief one, a career during which he or she can analyse only a limited number of candidates; and this tendency is heightened by the fact that in a significant number of training facilities the number of candidates any one training analyst can have in analysis at a given time is prescribed administratively. [Weinshel 1982:434]

To be a newly graduated analyst implies finding oneself standing on one of the lower rungs of the career ladder when one is some forty or fifty years old. It may then take an additional ten years before the analyst has found a voice of his own, and so a large number of analysts often conduct their most creative work when they are somewhere between fifty and sixty-five years old (King 1983:185): "You usually don't begin being a training analyst until you start to flirt with senility" (Weinshel interviewed in Raymond and Rosbrow-Reich 1997:201). To be able to embark upon a new career in late years may be a welcome impetus to personal development, but there will be the risk that those who are to tend to the varying aspects of training will form a rather aged crowd, which, one might suspect, is only lukewarmly intrigued by new and innovative ideas.

Around 1980, the share of training analysts among the world's graduate analysts (IPA) was 23 percent (Larsson 1982:382), and twenty years later the number was only marginally higher: 26 percent[7]: every fourth analyst, then, a number that witnesses to the fact that the status is both coveted and exclusive. "The psychoanalytic institute is not simply a training organization or a source of professional identification. Its activities constitute a particular form in which an analyst's career can be pursued, and its positions are prestigious attainments in the psychoanalytic world" (Dulchin and Segal 1982b:30). In some areas—especially in the United States, perhaps—this tendency has been so strong that "for many individuals there is a lingering sense of inferiority and incompletion which can be terminated only when they have achieved actualization of their unconscious fantasies of omnipotence in the form of an appointment as training analyst" (Arlow 1982:10; see also Arlow 1972:563).

Here lurks a serious problem in that psychoanalytic organizations on the whole lack the means of conveying recognition for psychoanalytical merit other than appointing someone as training analyst (officers within the IPA or its regional societies are most often already training analysts). The worst things about this are not the plausible compromises such that "training analysts may be appointed who may be popular and/or talented teachers or productive and/or prolific paper writers who may not, however, be top-notch analysts" or that "highly competent clinical analysts may not be called as training analysts because they are lack-lustre or ineffective teachers or have not made palpable contributions to our scientific literature" (Weinshel 1982:442). The real danger lies in its engendering a class system with dire consequences for life in psychoanalytic organizations.

Even if there is a board or specific committees for handling the appointment of training analysts, the institution of the training analyst as such is not a formal structure. Cremerius has pointed out how the democratic institutions within psychoanalytic societies—which, from a formal point of view, would be sovereign—often are totally lacking in influence when it comes to appointing training analysts (1987:1079). In addition, the appointments are often more oriented along political lines rather than those of clinical proficiency—in a system where one gives support to one's own (previous) candidates and promotes their careers within the institute. Not seldom will these processes take place outside of formal channels and without any means of democratic control over what criteria for selection have been utilized (Kernberg 1986:805). In this way, the group of training analysts tends to branch out around a lesser number of central figures who, by political means, have seen to it that "their" candidates will be favored within the training system. In brief: "Educational committees perpetuate themselves" (Aarons 1982–1983:679).

In that way, the training analyst institution will easily become an aristocratic club for mutual admiration, which will put its members in "a position that carries with it the connotation of 'superiority.'" (Aarons:679). To this group of phenomena belong the kind of considerations which are not unusual and whose essential aim is to keep track of who in the line of descendance stands closest to Freud: whose training analyst has been in analysis with whom, who in his turn. . . to finally land with The Great Master. The "right" and most "superior" training analyst is the one who can show the smallest amount of interjacent generations: "The importance of the genealogical tree became clear to me when I took on functions in the committees of the IPA. When the qualification of applicants from countries where there was as yet no recognized group were examined, more note was taken of the training analyst's position in the genealogy than of the qualification" (Thomä 1993:50).

The bundle of divergent interests and hidden procedures so often lying behind an appointment as training analyst is hardly conducive to the efficacy of the organizations and also contributes to the fact that in the psychoanalytic world "power does not come via the expression of an individual talent . . . it comes via the accrual of status in an insular and labyrinthine social network. The stages of achievement here consist very largely in the passing of time under critical scrutiny by authority figures" (Frosch 1997:6).

"It is disturbing but true that most [institutional] conflicts have originated over who shall have the right to train, that is, who shall be training analyst. The tensions emanating from the division of colleagues into two categories of analysts, training analysts and just plain analysts, intrude themselves into the organizational and scientific life of the institutes" (Arlow 1972:559). This problem not only affects the institute's task of providing education, but to a greater extent the body of psychoanalysts as a whole, as they are forced to live with a class system with severe social effects and not so few individual tragedies:

> [A] psychoanalyst, about 50 years old, had been an energetic enthusiastic society member. He . . . decided to apply for membership in the institute. He was treated coldly and critically, and, although his skills were at least equal to those of the average institute member, he was rejected for unconvincing reasons. He could not accommodate such behavior within the scope of what he saw good analysis to be. He withdrew from the society to his own practice, which he continued to enjoy, but never again participated in any society meetings, business or scientific. He was left permanently disillusioned with the quality of behavior of his colleagues, as well as profoundly angry and hurt. This is not uncommon. [Greben 1982–1983:662–663]

Conditions are not much different in Europe. The following story comes from the British Society:

> Only very recently, I happened to meet someone, an extremely good clinician, who hadn't openly done, as you might say, a great deal for psychoanalysis. She is a very independent person and hadn't been known to settle on either side of the Society's divide. Well into her fifties, she had applied for the second time to be made a training analyst, and was again turned down . . . which suggests to me that the wrong people are doing the selection, and that their selective powers are creaking. [Coltart, quoted in Molino 1997:178][8]

Now, power is not always sweet to the palate. Electing candidates and appointing new training analysts is often a burdensome process to those involved. It not only has to do with the insecurity involved when passing judgment that will have far-reaching consequences, but also with choosing and rejecting among colleagues and sometimes even among friends (see Orgel 1982). To become a training analyst is to change from being a clinician to also being

an evaluator of (future) colleagues: "Many training analysts com-
plain about their rigorous role and its strain on them. They point
out that everything conspires to turn the training analyst into a
master despite himself" (Dorn 1969:244).

> Some members find this very difficult and feel that the judg-
> mental aspect of the training analyst's role is antithetical to psy-
> choanalysis. This causes a serious identity crisis for some
> training analysts, which they never seem to resolve. Others
> respond to this identity crisis by becoming "Bolshie" and a "law
> unto themselves," refusing to work within training procedures
> and eventually breaking away from the psychoanalytic soci-
> ety. [King 1989:345]

Incestuous Ties, Oedipal Relations, and Power

No father would analyse his son, but something like this
happens in the training analysis.
                    —R. Bernardi and M. Nieto 1992:141

The wish to mould a man in one's own image is so
ubiquitous that not even God is exempt from it; it is a
manifestation of primary narcissism with which our
educational system is too much imbued.
                    —N. Nielsen 1954:249

Within the social connections that arise around the training analyst institution and the training institutes, a peculiar propensity
for developing family-like relationships can be met with. In fact,
such relationships seem to be the very form in which the psychoanalytic institution seeks to relieve itself of the tensions and problems that issue from its class system, while at the same time they
are symptoms of just this state of affairs. And, just as is characteristic of family relationships, there is a high level of intimacy,
and simultaneous with that, distinct limits between different categories of members.

In Chapter 4 I questioned the notion that identification would be the primary basis for a candidate acquiring positive or wished-for qualities and functions from his training analyst or supervisor. However, when it comes to the narcissistic ties that perhaps unavoidably arise between training analyst and candidate it does seem apt to speak in terms of identificatory processes, as these seem to be connected with different forms of dependency, both in the sense that they tend to arise within dependency relationships and that the identification as such engenders a (narcissistic) dependency on the chosen model, who will continue to be needed for the maintenance of the identification.

Considering the circumstances, the candidate's tendency to identification is understandable, although also problematic. More surprising, though, is the tendency of institutes to contribute to such processes. And here we are dealing with something much more obvious on the part of the training analyst than just his institutional role. It has to do with *the training analyst's* (or, just as well, the supervisor's) *identification with the candidate*: "While the candidate looks to the training analyst as a model for his own future as an analyst, the analyst sees in the candidate his professional offspring" (Shapiro 1976:31). In this way, an important aspect of the training analyst's countertransference will be his "unconscious or conscious tendency to *foster the candidate's identification with him, his dependence on him*" (Benedek 1954:15, italics in original). The result of this is that the training analyst will often become overprotective of his candidate and he may, for example, react to criticisms aimed at the candidate as if they were personal insults aimed at himself. Benedek ascribes this overprotection to a feeling of insufficiency on the part of the training analyst, as if he had promised too much and made the candidate expect to become a totally happy and free individual who, on top of it all, is an excellent analyst. But because no one knows how such things come about or how the result would look, uncertainty prevails.

Free discussion of candidates is like parents discussing their children; family rivalries take on an all too real aspect, and not

even training analysts are proof against battling for their
favorite children. In other words, the analyst is no longer a de-
tached participant observer—he has taken his stake in his
candidate's fate and some power to manipulate it. [Thompson
1958:48]

Dorn writes that "a training analysis evokes [in the analyst] powerful parenting-like forces, with an associated sense of self-
righteousness, rationalizing intrusiveness, and a need to know
about colleagues' inner lives" (1982–1983:694). He mentions these
kinds of feelings as a possible background to the fact that even
experienced analysts have been enrolled in different forms of
reporting systems.

The training analyst's difficulties in containing his countertransference—more specifically his narcissistic investment in his
candidates' analyses being successful (Greenson 1967:3; Kairys
1964:493)—may lead to exaggerated ambitions for the candidates
to evidence good results both clinically and intellectually. Nacht
speaks of the training analyst's wish to guide "his" candidate
toward a "brilliant success" (Nacht 1954:252). Because he feels
compelled to get as many of his candidates as possible "through"
he might also be tempted to influence the training system's evaluation of his analysand and—something which is not least grave—
perhaps to retain his loyalty far beyond the termination of the
training analysis (Greenacre 1966:555). For, as Weigert points out,
"Not only the analysand needs the analyst's acceptance, the analyst needs the analysand's genuine acceptance as well" (1955:638).

Among analysts, together with these "parental worries," there
is often also a striking anxiety that candidates will not be aware
of their proper place and position. King (1989:341) has pointed
out how analytical training programs tend at first to disrobe the
candidate of whatever professional identity he may have had
before entering training; he is not really allowed to establish a new
one before he has undergone a protracted period of trials where
all is uncertain as to whether he shall make the grade, so to speak,
until the very end. Leaning upon analytical theories that wish to

underscore the need for the child to realize and accept the distance between the generations (so it will not develop a perverse personality organization), we gladly speak of the candidates being in need of support in maintaining a "realistic" view of their position in the "succession of generations," despite the fact that in our day candidates and their teachers often belong to the same age group. It is as if we had some difficulty in discerning, on the one hand, the difference between knowing and experience, and on the other the difference between children and adults.

The candidate's ambition to become a member of the same profession as his analyst is, of course, an exceedingly important fact demanding special observance, especially as one considers the processes of identification. Because the candidate is a potential rival, it is in the analyst's interest to "have the candidate on his side" (Thompson 1958:49). And, as has been observed by Weinshel, in addition to the candidate's fantasies and wishes may be added such components as "identifying with, competing with, and ultimately succeeding the training analyst" (1982:439). Orgel inquires: "Is there any analysis in which the analyst is not at least partly a Lear awaiting the fate of being killed by the children?" (1990:10). The candidate's wish to (symbolically) murder the training analyst by replacing him will give rise to fantasies concerning the latter's need of revenge—thus "his expected criticism is anxiously circumvented by the candidate and he is constantly suspected of hostile reactions which may destroy the candidate's training opportunity" (Anna Freud quoted in Bibring 1954:169).

> The training analyst should encourage the analysand to question the analyst's omnipotence and to overtake and, in some ways, surpass the father-analyst. Many training analysts do not do this because of the unconscious fantasy of being devalued and destroyed by the son. Instead the analysand is rewarded for compliance, agreement, and admiration. [Greben 1982–1983:662]

To the extent that transference and countertransference reactions of this kind remain unanalyzed in candidates or acted out on the part of training analysts, precisely those kinds of relations that seem to characterize psychoanalytic conglomerations ever since their inception will establish themselves: "a 'family situation' where sibling rivalry and continuing transferences to the representations of authority are subtly encouraged" (Shapiro 1976:30). Sibling rivalry will lay the groundwork for severely competitive groups with strong tendencies toward collective acting out, controlling each other's progress, and comparing achievements.

> Less experienced analysts, especially students, find themselves in a milieu in which awe and reverence . . . are displaced onto training analysts; fulfilling, as they do, parental roles of acceptance or rejection. This state of affairs is a hangover from the period of candidacy, turning "fratricidal" among colleagues competing for the achievement of training analyst status. [Aarons 1982–1983:680; see also Bibring 1954:170; Greenacre 1966:554–556]

In this connection, one will often read of "convoying," a term coined by Greenacre to designate the kind of coterie of loyal followers that certain training analysts have been able to cultivate. Aarons describes the candidate's motive for joining such a group as "the transference [always leaving] a sequela of an affiliation bias favoring adherence to one's analyst in which what is accepted as authoritative in psychoanalytic development becomes so by virtue of the authoritarian role invested in the training analyst" (1982–1983:681).[9]

The identificatory ties between analyst and candidate may give rise to the former's "concern about the success of the student's analysis as reflecting on the analyst who analyzed him, preoccupation with the judgment of colleagues, using students in struggles against rivals in the field, over-identifying with the candidate as against the faculty or administration, excessive benevolence to insure having satellites, 'convoying' the analysand, etc." (Shapiro 1976:24). In this way are established—within narcissistically colored dependency relations—extremely strong demands for loyalty, either to the theoretical school to which the leader himself adheres, or to the theoretical doctrine he created.

Ties may grow so strong that the only way of liberating oneself is to revolt (see, for example, Kairys 1964:487). With these "unhealthy identifications and unresolved ambivalent transferences" one often seeks to explain what is commonly named "deviant theories and practices" (Greenacre 1966:548).

Heimann writes that "the dangers for the training analyst lie in his *temptation to modify* his technical procedure" (1954:164, italics in original). One may suspect, for example, that issues cropping up in the transference of a training analysis and having a basis in the reality of the institute shared by both may run the risk of being passed by in silence, as the requirement that the analyst remain "neutral" will easily paralyze him in such situations (Thomä 1993:43). The risk of deviations taking place is probably greatest in connection with the candidate's negative transference, that is to say, his hate. Negative transference is always difficult for both parties to handle and it should be no surprise that it could be more trying in cases when the the two run the risk of one day becoming colleagues: "When the negative transference has not been satisfactorily worked through, analysands will introject an unrealistic image of the training analyst which will serve as the kernel both of a new superego formation and for the organization of a pathological-narcissistic identification" (Cremerius 1987:1074). Problems of this kind place a special demand on the personal integrity of the training analyst.[10]

THE SUPEREGO COMPLEX

What we consciously intend to achieve with our candidates, is that they should develop a strong critical ego, capable of bearing considerable strains, free from any unnecessary identification, and from any automatic transference or thinking patterns. Contrary to the conscious aim our own behaviour as well as

the working of the training system have several features leading necessarily to a weakening of these ego functions and to
the formation and strengthening of a special kind of super-ego.
[Balint 1948:167]

The Immanent Pedagogy of the Psychoanalytic Institution

We have seen several examples of how one seeks the explanation for analysts' complex relations with one another, with their
organizations, and with psychoanalysis itself—"Envy, rivalry,
power conflicts, the formation of small groups, resulting in discord
and intrigues, are a matter of course" (Van Der Leeuw 1968:161)—
in unresolved transferences (see, for example, Weigert 1955:634ff).
The usual overrating of the training analysis—as if it were the only
really important part of training—comes to the fore in how its
shortcomings are deplored: "Transference residues result from
incomplete analyses so that conflicts become, and after the termination of the analysis remain, organized around the person and
image of the analyst" (Pfeffer 1963:243). I do not in any way wish
to dismiss such explanations, but I do perceive them as somewhat
simplified, not least because they seem to be repeated like a refrain or mantra. The complicated relationships between psychoanalysts must be considered in a larger context having to do with
the institute, its pedagogy and view of the candidates, and, finally,
with the training analyst institution as such.

The training curriculum and affiliation with a professional
group can be viewed as a gradually progressing process of socialization or acculturation (see Buechler 1988). Psychoanalytic training is a radical experience to most, and Zinberg writes that "some
of the values that develop during psycho-analytic candidacy, and
which in part perhaps conflict with previous values, become aspects of our identities as analysts and, in a sense, our way of life"
(1967:88). The value system and identity formation mentioned by
Zinberg can be problematic, for, as Arlow has pointed out, "the
guiding principles of the psychoanalytic curriculum do not always

correspond to the neatly phrased paragraphs bravely set in the pages of the institute's brochure or catalog" (1982:5). Apart from the qualities and skills that are required for the practice of psychoanalysis and that the training is meant to transmit and refine, there is often a learning process of a much darker nature. I am here talking about structurally determined effects arising outside the horizon of explicit aims and motives. In the language of Per-Johan Ödman, we can call this an *immanent pedagogy*,[11] a phenomenon that in no way is limited to psychoanalytic organizations, but seems to breed everywhere that people with strong common interests gather in sufficient numbers:

> No educational institution teaches just through its courses, workshops, and institutes; no corporation teaches just through its in-service education programs; and no voluntary organization teaches just through its meetings and study groups. They all teach by everything they do, and often they teach opposite lessons in their organizational operation from what they teach in their educational program. [Knowles 1973:100]

By definition, a pedagogy that is immanent exists outside the realm of what is openly stated and immediately visible. To capture its nature, when investigating what we take to be its effects, we need an interpretive stance together with a guiding hypothesis. The guiding hypothesis in this case is the heuristic concept of the psychoanalytical superego complex, which, as we have seen, is thought of as consisting of the professional superego and the institutional superego system. One starting point for my account is that it is the immanent pedagogy that lays the groundwork for this superego complex. We should therefore regard the complex not primarily as the expression of the strivings of particular individuals or groups, but as an effect of structural conditions.

To clear a path into this area I will start with a short theoretical exposition on my own view of the nature of the superego and the ego ideal, their dynamics and ways of functioning. Being theoretical entities, superego and ego ideal are instruments for a heuristic approach to the phenomena at hand; in no way do they designate empirical "facts." Part of the discussion concerning the ego ideal will come in this section; part will be saved for the end of this chapter.

This will be a rather condensed presentation of the concepts as I define them. On the whole I abstain from giving an account of their origins and development and also of my own deviations from established usage after Freud. It would simply be too unmanageable in this connection to insert a more far-reaching discussion of the conceptual definitions that I have chosen. Thus, I can only ask the reader to accept the definitions presented and my use of the terms *superego* and *ego ideal* ad hoc et bona fide.

Superego and Ego Ideal

The concepts of ego ideal and superego both stem from Freud's article "On Narcissism" from 1914. From a strict point of view we only find the term "ego ideal," but the foundation for what is soon to come is already conceptually laid out, and is more or less complete. He writes: "It would not surprise us if we were to find a special psychical agency which performs the task of seeing that narcissistic satisfaction from the ego ideal is ensured and which, with this end in view, constantly watches the actual ego and measures it by that ideal" (Freud 1914a:95). Such an authority, which can observe and criticize the subject's intentions, is known from everyday life: it is called "the conscience," a term Freud appoints as the guardian to ensure that the ego ideal is really being obeyed. And it is the obeying of this ideal that is the basis for the feeling that Freud here emphasizes: *Selbstgefühl*, self-esteem.

In the article "Mourning and Melancholia" from 1917, the ego ideal as such is not mentioned, only the conscience. Freud makes a comparison between the processes at hand within the subject when in a state of mourning and what occurs in states of melancholia or deep depression. In the mourner, all attention is gathered around the lost Other, and he will experience the world as empty and meaningless. As for the melancholic, his own ego stands in the foreground, and here it is the *inner* world that has become a wasteland: "The patient represents his ego to us as worthless, incapable of any achievement and morally despicable; he reproaches himself, vilifies himself and expects to be cast out and punished. He abases himself before everyone and commiserates with his own relatives for being connected with anyone so unworthy" (Freud 1917:246). In melancholy, says Freud, it is as if that part of the ego he calls the conscience sets itself above another part and makes of it an *object* to be criticized and condemned.

In the seventh chapter of "Group Psychology and the Analysis of the Ego," from 1921, Freud gives a sweeping reference to his account from 1917, and the self-observing and critical instance—conscience—is now suddenly and without any comment placed on equal footing with the ego ideal. In all we can see, it is quite apparent that to Freud it is still a matter of the same ego ideal as he presented in the article on narcissism in 1914. And, with the advent of "The Ego and the Id," published in 1923, the terminology is again somewhat displaced. What previously had been known as ego ideal now finds competition from another concept: "the superego." And without any apparent inconvenience, Freud now uses the two terms interchangeably, as if in fact they were equivalents.

The superego is directly connected with Freud's theory of the Oedipus complex and its dissolution: that is to say that chain of events when the child abandons its incestuous wishes directed toward the parent of the opposite sex. The authority—the father's, the mother's, or that of society—exacting this sacrifice from the child is internalized in an identificatory process and *"confronts the other contents of the ego as an ego ideal or super-ego"* (Freud 1923b:34, italics in original). The ego ideal (or superego) "answers to everything that is expected of the higher nature of man" (1923b:37). Freud is referring to its function as the locality of our moral sense and conscience. The subject's experience of guilt arises in the tension that can occur between the demands of conscience and the empirical ego's actual deeds.

To Freud, the ego ideal would in many senses remain a transitional concept on the way to the more comprehensive superego, which then would contain both a prohibiting aspect and a guiding aspect following from the appropriation of an ideal. In "The Ego and the Id," he uses the terms without any distinction, only to subsume the ideal later, in the "New Introductory Lectures on Psycho-Analysis" (1933), as a mere component function within the more encompassing superego.

My view is that we should regard Freud's arrangement of the ego ideal under the superego as an attempt to combine incompatible entities. In what follows, I maintain that there is a decisive difference between ego ideal and superego that makes it impossible to subsume them under the same category. I find that two wholly different kinds of affective energy seem to be active in the respective "metabolisms":[12] the superego operates by subjugating its object, the ego, utilizing the latter's fear—whereas submission under the ego ideal is an act of love as the subject seeks to correspond to its (chosen) model. (In a later section of this chapter, "The Psychoanalyst's Inner Career," I will have more to say about the ego ideal.)

Fueled by Hate

Freud characterizes the superego as an instance with a "compulsive character which manifests itself in the form of a categorical imperative" (Freud 1923b:35). The inexorability of the superego becomes even more obvious in "Civilization and Its Discontents," where he writes that "the more virtuous a man is, the more severe and distrustful is its behaviour, so that ultimately it is precisely those people who have carried saintliness furthest who reproach themselves with the worst sinfulness" (Freud 1930:125–126). To Freud, the superego is the introjected representative of an external authority, and the subject's continued sacrifices that aim at satisfying its demands can only lead to its being strengthened and becoming even more strict. The superego expects obedience, but will never settle for what it gets, and continues to unrelentingly torment even the most virtuous individual. In Freud's description, man is inescapably prisoner to the superego.

In "Beyond the Pleasure Principle," from 1920, Freud abandoned his previous theory of the drives and introduced a new categorization, this time dividing them between the life instincts and the death (or destructive) drive. To Freud the death drive is the superego's primary instinctual source. For example, in melancholia, where an implacable superego rages at the ego, showering it with criticism and reproaches, there rules "a pure culture of the death instinct" (1923b:53). It is not until he has presented his theory of this death drive that the superego finally is depicted as so totally inexorable. Earlier, he had certainly described how it can harass and torment the ego, but the theory had no conception of its inexorability as a constant force.

The death drive is for Freud a kind of biological principle that pushes the living organism toward its own extinction and at the same time attaches itself to the other drives, making them "conservative" in the sense that they are made to cling to already established forms and oppose change. When this death drive is projected toward the outer world it will appear as aggressiveness and the pure destructiveness that comes to the fore in, for example, man's endless wars. But one may well ask how a biological tendency for the organism's physiological self-destruction can be grasped in psychological or, even better, affective terms.[13] Rather than a death drive, I would therefore prefer to speak of *hate* as a primary psychic source of energy together with the *libido*, which Freud spoke of as the instinctual source of love. Hate is recognizable as a human phenomenon and is a category that does not rest upon questionable pseudobiological speculation; it is furthermore not dependent upon the unconvincing mechanics of projection that a death drive must undergo for it to become plausible as aggressivity or destructivity.

Hate is a component aspect of the fundamental patterns of the subject's relation with the world, and crystallizes primarily as the impulse to destroy what is Other (i.e., that which is foreign) or *the* Other, my fellow human being, who not only frustrates my desires and needs but also invades me, puts demands on me, and leaves me with a surplus of stimuli. Just like the libido, hate is a force looking for an object. It clusters in different states of density related to specific objects, which can be the Other, the Other's Being, or the Other's desire. Only when hate has connected with an object is it possible for the subject, through introspective scrutiny, to recognize it as a discernible affect, "feeling," or sentiment—as hatred.[14]

Anyone alive will have experience of how the superego may haunt the ego whenever it for some reason has been weakened—the ego's failures or mishaps even seem to spur the superego's fervent hate. Perhaps the most cruel form of such trials is melancholy, where the superego ravages the ego full blast. In this there is no pardon when the subject is exposed to a torrent of attacks whose undermining message wedges into every crevice of consciousness to spread its poison of self-hatred and self-contempt. In this tyranny of the superego there is something inexorable, like an insatiable drive that will show itself as soon as the opportunity arises. When it is not turned against the self but externalized, the same hate will eagerly seek an object in the outer world.

Hate is, of course, a close neighbor to love, and they demonstrate some similarities, both surprising and terrifying. Freud said of love's instinctual energy that it is afflicted with a degree of "adhesiveness," making it reluctant to let go of objects once chosen. Even though the fact was never pointed out by Freud, the same seemingly applies to hate, which will frequently evolve into an ardent passion, a symptomatic madness that tends to bind the subject in a common fate with a fellow human being or sometimes a social institution or even an idea. He also wrote of the ego as a reservoir of libido (1905:218)—not the *source* of the libido, but a place where it is "stored" and perhaps also "managed." In line with this, I would like to proclaim the superego as the reservoir for introjected hate.

The Superego Complex as the Culture of Hate

In the previous chapter we discussed internalization as the absorption and transformation of intersubjective relationships into subjective structures. Lebovici has pointed out that "the training analyst hands down a heritage, not only by the quality of his analytical work with candidates, but also by his own work, his scientific and cultural interests, not to mention his character" (1978:135). "Candidates will tend to introject the handling of power allocation and other ethical qualities of the interpersonal relations in the institute onto their psychoanalytic ego ideal and superego" (Stensson 1993:53), and to the extent that the training analyst institution is characterized by enactment of power, control, and rivalry, interaction with the institute will result in negative internalizations. Thus "concepts of power and violence may then become part of the student's ego ideal, and fear rather than love would be central" (Dorn 1969:242).

Of all the viewpoints that may be applied to the immanent pedagogy of psychoanalytic training, hate would certainly be the most fateful one when it comes to the transmission of the professional superego. From that vantage point, what has been touched upon here by Lebovici, Stensson, and Dorn is all about the transmission of hate between analytic generations. It is the professional superego that functions as a reservoir for the hate internalized through the immanent pedagogy described here. This superego is no new or separate structure within the personality, but an extension of the superego that every individual has been endowed with during his formative years.

Our more surveyable social interactions (as, for example, pair relations, families, smaller groups, and, not least important in this connection, the psychoanalytic pair) seem to have a certain advantage when it comes to their developing in an atmosphere of love and care. (That is one reason we more often allow ourselves to ventilate our anger at home rather than at work, where the threat of retribution is considerably more severe.) It is more evident how larger groups and organizations tend to be marked by a more or less prominent culture of hate. Although I hope to demonstrate the function of the professional superego as a juncture for this culture within psychoanalytical organizations, for other social systems and groups we may as yet only hypothesize that such an instance is in effect there as well.

That smaller social structures would be conducive to a culture of care and that hate tends to agglutinate within larger ones may at least in part be explained by the fact that within smaller and surveyable contexts ethical sensibility has a stronger position (hate is thereby not absent, but more effectively contained and sublimated).[15] I will not venture into a discussion of how, for example, family structures and surrounding social contexts may contribute to the development and sustenance of an ethical frame of mind, but will restrict myself to simply asserting that this is the case. Conversely, the tendency of hate to put its mark upon relations within most larger social structures would seem to be directly connected with the ethical frame of mind not being equally vigilant. On the level of larger groups and organizations, as in society itself,[16] we are instead guided by legal and deontological frames, which is to say some kind of written or interpersonally sustained set of rules for conduct. Whether one should take this to be an "eternal and unavoidable" complication will have to be an issue for ethical philosophy.

To conclude: the superego complex is a heuristic instrument for exploring a system and an inner dynamic underlying how certain destructive factors are transmitted within psychoanalytic institutes and societies. The complex may be said to be played out on the interface between the professional superego and the institutional superego system, where each supplies the other with their respective contents, forms, and energies. The professional superego is that form in which the hate invested in the institutional superego system is individually introjected through the immanent pedagogy of the training system and other organizational forms. Conversely, the superego system is that form in which the professional superego's reservoir of introjected hate is externalized and allowed to take form institutionally. To the complex thus established, hate, in the interchange between superego and superego system, will function as an affective "glue" allowing the complex to survive coherently over time.[17]

King expresses a similar thought as she writes that the psychoanalytic institution becomes "an extension of themselves, and their ego structures become parasitical on it" (1983:188). If we add the psychoanalyst's professional superego to the ego structures mentioned by King we meet with an image of the interdependency between individual and institutional structures. On this issue Rangell writes that the superego "serve[s] as a bridge between the individual and the group" (1974:8).

It should be underlined that the processes I address here under the rubric of a superego complex differ from the "primitive" processes taken by many as an example of the tendency of groups to allow regressive patterns to evolve. In such cases it is often a question of the group's tendency to create inner tensions while at the same time reducing individual control, as, for example, when there is a case of mobbing or sexual transgression. Apart from the individual and specific manifestations of such a dynamic, it may also become established in the form of corrupted and corrupting patterns of behavior, which could include subgroups tolerating (and feeding upon) consistent sabotage of all attempts to reform or better an organization, late arrivals, tardiness in work presentation, or theft of available materials as an accepted expression of tacit dissatisfaction and hate. Even if these behaviors evolve into developed and stable "cultures" within, for example, a division of an organization, the patterns of behavior remain dystonic, in the sense that they might be defended by a perpetrator when directly confronted, but not without visible signs of shame.

My immediate interest centers, however, upon a phenomenon that is considerably more structured. The hate animating the superego complex is not something that spurts out in instances when the institution or group loses its grip on the direction of the work it is supposed to perform and/or loses its capacity to contain the impulses of its members, but is rather an integrated (and definitely deplorable) aspect of the way of organizing the psychoanalytical institution during the third epoch. The superego complex—in contradistinction to the dystonic patterns just mentioned—has a clearer syntonic character. In this chapter and the previous one there are several examples to substantiate how it is possible for its defenders to unabashedly stand up for different aspects of the whole complex (if not for the hate that makes the whole thing go round).

Externalized Hate

Freud spoke, as we have seen, of the evolution of the superego as a process of identification involving the introjection of external authority. On that very point Anna Freud has developed a theory of specific interest to our study of the transformations of the professional superego. She writes of an "identification with the aggressor" as an early stage in the development of the superego and also as a stage in the paranoid process (1936). Identification with the aggressor takes place in the form of accepting and introjecting the critical voice of the Other (which now becomes "my own"), while at the same time the "crime" that the critical voice would condemn is projected upon the outer world. Result: "*They* are the guilty ones, not I." Through this externalization the subject hopes to avoid the sense of guilt issuing from a conflict with the superego.

Arlow writes: "It is unfortunate that, educationally speaking, the most reliable method for achieving identification is to treat the individual cruelly" (1982:13). It is not that the analytical training program is overtly cruel, but it is in all probability more demanding, more controlling, and more strict than many other educational systems: "Analytic training is frustrating and, in some ways, even demeaning" (Weinshel 1982:437). The institutional severity of psychoanalytic training makes it easy to understand that "masochistic submission would appear to be the most common posture assumed by the candidate" (Dorn 1969:251). Masochistic submission may be the easiest and simplest path to adaptation, but it does also open the doors for identification with the aggressor.

Anna Freud describes how she could observe in a boy of six how he apparently did not identify with the person of the aggressor, but with aggression as such (1936:112). This observation is important for our discussion, for it gives a good illustration of my use of the term *internalization*. For internalization as the assimilation of intersubjective relations and their transformation into subjective structures pertains—just as with the boy—precisely to *the appropriation of a way of being* rather than the emulation of a model.

When the candidate graduates and becomes an analyst he is no longer merely the recipient of the immanent pedagogy of hate, but in his different roles and functions he is also the keeper of the hate that he has introjected to form his superego and thus made his own. In a process similar to what Anna Freud calls identification with the aggressor, the internalized and terrorizing hate can then be deflected from the ego and directed toward the outer world. Then it will manifest itself in more or less subtle personal attitudes or institutional forms, as when giving support to strict rules and the control of candidates and/or colleagues, subtle processes of ejection, theoretical and clinical orthodoxy, and so on.

In this way hate is transmitted between psychoanalytic generations, and as a result there follows a tendency for paranoization of the relations within analytic professional organizations. As with the transmission of hate in a dialectical reproductive circuit moving between an internalized superego and an institutional superego system, paranoia issues from the very structures it has given rise to. Within this sphere there are no direct connections, and for that reason it is impossible for me to offer a general description that moves from causes to their effects. The superego complex stands out as a network of mutually interacting factors and forces that at the same time both support and breed one another. Thus it would be erroneous to claim that this kind of social phenomenon is *caused* by hate, but it certainly does tap the superego's reservoir of hate for a vital part of the energy it needs for its existence.

Paranoia, Hostility, and the Pursuit of the Psychopath

Let us now take a look at how transmission of the kind mentioned can take place by examining the hush-hush that so often prevails within psychoanalytic institutes. Kernberg ascribes "the paranoid atmosphere that often pervades psychoanalytic institutes and its devastating effect on the 'quality of life' in psychoanalytic education" (1986:803), among other things, to the institutes' notorious lack of ability to or interest in codifying in clear and precise terms what is required of the candidate. It is rather the rule that the general demands and norms or (negative or positive) opinions coming from supervisors or teachers and underlying the decisions taken by the institute on behalf of individual candidates—be it a question of selection, the evaluation of progress, graduation, or expulsion—are only summarily or selectively accounted for, if at all.

> There is a group of officials—more particularly the training analysts—which like parents negotiate behind locked doors and are allowed to keep their discussions and decisions secret: access to training, to the preliminary seminars and the seminars has not been discussed—and is in most places still not discussed—openly with the candidates. They have no influence upon the curriculum nor on the educational content. [Cremerius 1987:1068]

Weiss writes that when a candidate who is felt to be problematic—which could be anything from his being oppositional to really detrimental to his analysands—is finally confronted with a final decision on the part of the institute it often turns out that he has been ignorant of his situation having been perceived as problematic (1982:80). One important reason for the lack of information reaching candidates is that the decisions are often based upon information that is difficult to reveal openly, at times even between the decision makers themselves:

> The social structure of a psychoanalytic training institute displays a unique system of communication. Its distinctiveness derives from the fact that its senior members acquire a kind of knowledge about all members of the institute that the superordinates of no other organization gather about their members—the information and understandings generated through psychoanalysis. Senior members not only analyze their students and junior colleagues but also make the administrative decisions which govern the careers of these junior members. . . . The decisions which the senior members make about such matters are based not only on impressions and evaluations acquired from direct encounters with junior colleagues, graduates and students. The desire to base their decisions upon the most comprehensive knowledge leads senior members to use other kinds of information, including confidential information derived from the analyses of both junior members and of people who know them who are in analysis privately with the senior members of the institute. [Dulchin and Segal 1982b:27]

That the analysand speaks as openly and candidly as possible with his analyst is one of the fundamental precepts of the analytic dialogue. When the analysand is expected to speak of everything that comes to mind in the form of ideas and emotions, even a self-imposed censorship as to the identity of persons mentioned will often become the target for interpretations in terms of resistance or avoidance. In this way an analyst will accrue considerable amounts of information, not only concerning his own analysands but also on a great many people in their surroundings.

Under "normal" circumstances this may not pose a major problem for the analysands, their acquaintances, or the analysts themselves. But it is easy to appreciate what the effect may be when so many of those involved in these informational networks are active within one and the same social context, as is the case in a psychoanalytical society or institute, where "not only . . .

all institute members undergo analysis with at least one of the senior members, but also some relatives, friends and outside colleagues of institute members undergo analysis by the same senior analysts" (Dulchin and Segal 1982b:29).[18]

Training analysts themselves are hardly exempt from being scrutinized in this network of informal information processing. Because a candidate's supervisor functions as the analyst of another one, within the group of training analysts as a whole a substantial amount of knowledge going crosswise in all directions will evolve, with the candidates as the system's (most often) ignorant and innocent messengers. In this way it is possible to evaluate the competence of colleagues who wish to become training analysts, and to some extent even tap available information and judgments concerning one's own person, not only among colleagues but also among those one happens to supervise.

Thus is formed within the congregation of training analysts a "central intelligence agency," which covers not only candidates and a large group of their acquaintances, but also the greater number of colleagues. Even if all involved were to be animated by the most impeccable integrity when it comes to handling confidential matters, the "sheltered" confidentiality makes it impossible to trace all this information that has been divulged in closed chambers back to its sources, which in turn makes it impossible to validate its relevance.

I wrote at the inception of this chapter that the phenomenon of the training analyst is more than just a class or caste system, and that it in fact constitutes an independent institution that does not conform to any formally structured organization. The divide between the training analyst institution and all the others—including both candidates and colleagues—is the very focal point of the psychoanalytic superego complex. Considering the information system involved with the training analyst institution, it is not difficult to imagine how a paranoid atmosphere may easily develop at the core of psychoanalytic collegiality, one that would manifest itself as a kind of obsessional suspicion about the mental health of colleagues, coupled with the worry that one may oneself be the object of such doubts. The process begins during the selection of candidates and has its final manifestation in the form of a collegiality characterized by hostility and fear, plus a phenomenon that I have chosen to designate as "the pursuit of the psychopath."

The pursuit of the psychopath is perhaps the most evident manifestation of how the persecutory element introjected with the professional superego can be projected against the outside world, whether that be the organization, theory, or the colleagues themselves. The pursuit seems in many quarters to have become a kind of specter haunting the analytic community and persevering in the form of a mainly subconscious but constant controlling and monitoring of what colleagues say, how they behave, and what is said about them. Here a worried and often subliminal search for some kind of fault is played out, which in this connection I choose to call "psychopathy," a diffusedly perceived disorder, an emotional perversion, which, if only it could be brought to the light of day, would merit the withdrawal of analytic certification. My use of the term "psychopathy" in this connection is in no way meant as a true diagnostic category, but rather functions as a code word for establishing disapproval or depreciation of both candidates and colleagues. It is actually not so rare in discussions between psychoanalysts (see, for example, Dulchin and Segal 1982a:17, 20, 21; also Kernberg 1986:831).

The pursuit begins, as we saw in the previous chapter, with the "advanced psychopathology" evidenced in the process of selection, where, according to Pollock, one often devotes "too much attention to studying failures, errors, or pathology" (1976:323). "We frequently feared that rather than being judged on our academic progress or our technical competence by objective criteria, we would be assessed according to our avowal of a particular analytic trend or the state of our personal pathology" (Bruzzone et al. 1985:411). The chase continues all through the training process, as institutes are inclined to interpret all the candidate's difficulties or conflicts with the institute and its representatives in terms of personal pathology: "questioning, doubting, criticizing on the part of candidates tends to be suspect" (Arlow 1970:11; see also Cremerius 1987:1087). The proposed solution is rather predictable: "Back to the couch!" In a fictitious and satirical guide for officials within a psychoanalytic training program Kernberg writes: "Refer all problems involving teachers and students, seminars and supervision, all conflicts between candidates and the faculty 'back to the couch'; keep in mind that transference acting out is a major complication of psychoanalytic training, and that there are always transference elements in all students' dissatisfaction" (1996:1038).

As the reverse of these exaggerated expectations for training analysis, the training analyst himself can be blamed for all of the candidate's shortcomings (Kernberg 1986:820). If it isn't the candidate who is deficient, the psychopath must, of course, be the analyst—in any case, he must be insufficiently analyzed (see Thomä 1993:57).

But, as is pointed out by Kernberg, one of the psychopath's distinctive characteristics is that he is so adept at hiding his psychopathy (1986:831). For that reason no one can ever be sure that the selection process or the training analysis has been effective enough to screen and reject him, and thus the suspicion lingers on that despite all precautionary measures, the superficially "normal" or "healthy" candidate has not been stopped from gaining access to the profession. Moral of the story: the psychopath may dwell anywhere in our midst.

Outside of the systems of education, the pursuit of the psychopath perseveres as a kind of institution in its own right. Van Der Leeuw writes that it is "much more difficult to acknowledge one's own motives and arguments than to express suppositions about the motives of others. Interpretation is frequently used between us as a weapon when questions of prestige are at stake" (1968:162). Arlow writes in the same vein of a "tendency to diagnose and label one's opponent rather than to understand his point of view. . . . Thus, those who disagree with the group are not considered to be misguided or perhaps slow in thought. There is something wrong with them" (Arlow 1970:10–11). Kernberg connects tendencies such as these to a kind of (unconscious) attempt to "transform the ideology of psychoanalytic institutes into a religious organization. . . . Psychoanalysis, in this transformation, is no longer a scientific theory to be continually reexamined, but a firmly established doctrine that also has an implied value as a *Weltanschauung*, a view of the world that readily explains the unconscious motives and resistances of those who do not agree with it" (1986:825).[19]

Beland (1983:52–54) depicts the psychoanalytic group identity as a force at once striving to attain consent, while at the same time inclined to exclusion. It strives for change, but at the same time its judgments are conservative. It is ahistorical and apolitical in its thinking and will gladly regard all fundamental insights and developments attained after the death of Freud as if they had been present within his thought from the beginning. The sense of identity becomes a matter of faith and dogma while doubt and criticism are anathema.

The paradoxical striving for consensus and its simultaneous will to exclude, which seem to characterize many psychoanalytical institutions (it has been compared with the processes within communist parties!), will effectuate the result we have identified as identification with the aggressor:

> Exclusion leads the excluded group to internalize the perspectives and standards of the excluding group, in a rigid and harsh way: a form of identification with the aggressor. Individuals in the excluded group come to believe that they don't measure up and that the values, standards, and points of view of the excluding group are the only legitimate ones. Alternative perspectives generated by members of the excluded group come to be thought of as inevitably, inherently inferior. The wish to emulate, and ultimately become a part of the excluding group can, and often does, become a powerful, almost obsessional motivator. [Slavin 1994:96–97]

A vicious circle establishes itself in which the excluding group (the training analysts) and the excluded (the rest) are united in a paradoxical alliance turned against everything that seems

to be unlike them. Arlow writes of how groups can develop that
are

> constantly concerned with the notion that analysis is threat-
> ened and has to be saved. Specifically they proclaim themselves
> as the defenders of Freud, determined to protect and to secure
> his priceless heritage and to transmit it intact and uncontami-
> nated. . . . The enemy, more often than not, is to be found
> within one's own institute or within the ranks of psychoanaly-
> sis. I have seen too often a recurrent tendency to separate the
> sheep from the goats, the "real analysts" from those who are
> not analysts at all. [1970:9][20]

If this way is established, according to our heuristic model, the
dialectic between institutional forms and the superego's stock of
hate, when externalized, contributes to the formation of antago-
nistic groups and to serious fissures, which in turn may be internalized by new generations as a professional superego.

The obvious difficulty of handling differences within the psychoanalytic community in an overt and generous way not only
has its effects on theory or the clinic, but—as an aspect of the
pursuit of the psychopath—also on a very personal level. He who
does not adhere to a conservative norm will often be the object of
a great deal of suspicion (see Greben 1982–1983:660).[21] This will,
for example, express itself in the nearly ubiquitous refusal to allow homosexuals to enter analytic training: "The justification for
such regulations is our 'knowing' that these people must, by definition, be as alleged: fatally flawed psychoticlike creatures in states
of near-annihilation of the self (covered over, of course, by nor-
mal-appearing behavior)" (Stoller 1985:182–183).

The awareness of this widespread intolerance has led some commentators, despite their good intentions of openness and tolerance,
to write what still seems a bit comical, when considering that the
issue itself should be rather self-evident: "There are persons who
do not achieve a balanced sexual life and who nevertheless do good
analytical work" (Van Der Leeuw 1962:281). Or: "It is theoretically
conceivable that specific, circumscribed areas of psychopathology

could, in a given candidate, facilitate his doing psychoanalytical work—a topic sorely in need of further theoretical elaboration and clinical documentation" (Calef and Weinshel 1980:281).

When it is a conscious and active attitude, the pursuit of the psychopath may be an activity within the mind in the form of more or less rapidly passing diagnostic and depreciating evaluations of colleagues. At its peak, the pursuit takes place in the closed chambers of discussion between trusted friends. But it does concern something beyond individual reflection and mere prejudice: it is an integral part of the power game among psychoanalysts, where it might not be as openly accounted for even by those who personally lead the chase as they decide upon graduations or election to a committee. Here the pursuit dissolves into a more nebulous force which, albeit to anyone concerned wholly tangible, will also color all social relations within the psychoanalytic community: hostility and fear.[22]

Grotstein writes about his experiences in the society where he was trained that "one of the most surprising discoveries to penetrate the immunity blanket of my naivete was the phenomenon of extraordinary hatred for each other among analysts" (1985:38). On the state of things within the British Society Coltart says: "Why not say that there are plenty of people in the Society who would appear perfectly amiable and friendly towards you while you were in the Society, but if the occasion arose, they would as soon stab you in the back?" (in Molino 1997:171–172). The matter is summarized by Van Der Leeuw when he writes that he has "the impression that there are few true friendships amongst our members" (1968:163; see also Greben 1982–1983:665–666). And, of course, in an organization characterized by hate and a paranoid atmosphere friendship *can* be dangerous.

The hate manifesting itself as hostility between colleagues will also affect candidates: "It is also this author's impression (from student days) that there may be much condescension and suppressed aggression that the training analyst has to restrain while with his analysands, but which he can let out on his supervisees" (Aarons 1982–1983:685). According to our fundamental hypothesis it is through the training—both with regard to its content and its forms—that hate is transmitted to the new generation through the inoculation of the psychoanalyst's professional superego with the immanent pedagogy. A kind of surplus effect follows such that to the extent that a superego is conveyed—and it is my contention that that is always the case—the leadership of the training body will, in the candidates' fantasies, be identified as rulers who hate their subjects.

The superego is not just an effect of life in professional organizations: internalized hate is part of human existence. Paranoia and hostility nurture the fear inculcated with the superego, the effect of which depends only on fear of the hateful rage that it can produce. It is not surprising, then, that fear will be a controlling affect in the collegial relations between analysts. Dulchin and Segal report that social intercourse at the institute where they had studied was characterized by anxiety, except in those who had reached the positions they had striven for. "Not knowing the uses to which confidences might be put, analysts tended to proceed with care and formality in conversation rather than throw caution to the winds and form relationships among their colleagues on more personal grounds. More often than not, everyday interactions among analysts were marked by a pattern of caution, lack of ease and even, at times, awkwardness" (1982b:36).[23]

In a short essay Klauber deplores the fact that "we know too little of what our colleagues really do" (1986:212). With the prohibiting aspect of the professional superego, an inner vigilant eye is installed that easily brings forth notions of criticism or condemnation from colleagues, should they have access to what goes on in one's own consulting room. The persistent thought that there are psychopaths among our ranks in a way presupposes its logical opposite: the normal individual and the perfect analyst (and what would be cause and effect here is difficult to say). The secrecy we touched on at the beginning of this section not only pertains to training institutes; life as a whole within psychoanalytic organizations is marked by it. The notion of the perfect analyst is the fantastic antipole to the psychopath. In this connection

Kernberg speaks of the ideal of a totally anonymous analyst, morally impeccable, without any outstanding personality traits, with a strong capacity for human understanding and lacking all convictions or opinions concerning everything else: "the man who pretends not to be God" (1986:818; see also Marmor 1953). To avoid the risk of being in any way less than this unattainable ideal the analyst—and the training analyst—is tempted to choose silence. There is also the fact that idealization of the analyst often seems to be left untouched in the training analyses (Greben 1982–1983:661), resulting in the "paranoization" of collegial relations with which we are already acquainted. Ultimately, it becomes difficult to share any of the more intimate aspects of the psychoanalytic experience at all.

> The analyst's use of humour is not often disclosed in formal presentations, but that is not to say that it does not occur. The paucity of literature on the subject is noteworthy and we might well conclude that this is an area where analysts prefer privacy, as in other areas where they might attract criticism from their colleagues, e.g., impasse, countertransference acting out, therapeutic failure, interminability, suicide, etc. [Baker 1993:952]

In an article on the relationship between psychoanalytic theory and practice Joseph Sandler writes:

> The idea that there might be a not-fully-integrated body of theory does not seem quite respectable. . . . It is my firm conviction that the investigation of the implicit, private theories of clinical psychoanalysts opens a major new door in psychoanalytic research. One of the difficulties in undertaking such research is that posed by the conscious or unconscious conviction of many analysts that they do not do 'proper' analysis (even though such a conviction may exist alongside the belief that they are better analysts than most of their colleagues). [1983:37–38][24]

The matter is in no way a new one, as exemplified by a speech given by the president of the APA in 1953: "I believe we may all be a little afraid that we are practicing analysis somewhat differ-

ently from the way others are doing it, and perhaps a little 'im-
properly' in terms of being less orthodox, introducing more modifications which we regard as necessary for the patients we treat,
and so on" (Knight 1953:219). There is a paranoid fear among
analysts to step forth and declare what they actually believe in
and how they think:

> Pressures toward theoretical conformity within an institute, for
> example, may be profound. It is not uncommon to see such
> phenomena as young graduate analysts who remain excessively
> deferential and constrained about speaking up at meetings, or
> who hold back from innovative and creative teaching or writ-
> ing, or who, despite good potential to develop in the field,
> somehow drift away. Providing opportunities to counteract
> such tendencies is especially crucial for the development of
> young faculty. [Fogel and Glick 1991:417]

Effects on Theoretical Work

In Chapter 2, theoretical work was emphasized as an important
aspect of the analyst's qualifications. Theoretical work is presumably the principal form for the way analysts engage in a dialogue
concerning the deeper aspects of the psychoanalytic experience. To
be sure, this applies also to the supervisory situation, but the clinical dialogue is, by necessity, limited to two persons or at least to
smaller groups and does not engender a wider discussion—supervision is, after all, more experience than reflection.

It was also stated that psychoanalytic knowing comprises three
levels: the experience that evolves in the the clinical encounter,
clinical theory, and metapsychology. Theoretical work is carried
out within all of these, but the kind of work that interests us in
this connection has to do with the construction of clinical theory
and metapsychological reflection. I make a distinction between
theoretical work and research. By the latter is most often understood varying forms of empirical investigations in a more accepted
scientific sense, such as studies on therapeutic efficacy, studies

covering the details of analytical processes, studies on the connection between psychoanalytic knowing and neuroscientific knowledge, and so forth. Less often, research will also be theoretical work or can at least include it as a component part.[25]

At its core, perhaps, theoretical work is an aspect of the analyst's mental preparation for the encounter with his analysand. This may be highlighted somewhat by Klauber's words that "the skills involved in the conceptualization of a paper are also highly important for doing good psychoanalysis" (1982–1983:678). Theoretical work becomes a necessity when a state of tension arises between the received mass of theory and the analyst's own clinical practice. The conflict has to be solved through reflection, and the road back to good analytical work will stop at such stations as the development of new ways of considering and understanding clinical experience, critique and evaluation of the existing theoretical tradition, or critique of the very metaphysical foundations upon which our knowledge rests.

> It is my conviction that the more urgent, the far more difficult need, and the larger potentiality for scientific and therapeutic progress lie in the constant examination and reexamination of our basic procedural assumptions and our related theories regarding psychoanalytic process and personality dynamics. It is in this sphere that, stated or unstated, the greatest resistance in the psychoanalytic community appears, and in a manner which to me, whether as general observer or as participant in discussion, betrays an unscientific (sometimes antiscientific) nonrational component. This I regard as the greatest single obstacle to the progress of psychoanalysis and as far more important than our selection of patients or even of candidates. . . . [Stone 1975:335–336]

With the excellent model of Freud's lifelong reevaluation of his own thoughts and precepts, psychoanalysis has been steadily changing, both in terms of its self-reflection in the form of theoretical discourse and in its clinical applications. Still, there have always been those who speak as if we were living in the best of worlds and that all the discoveries and theoretical formulations of psychoanalysis had already been made.[26] Analysts who view things from such an angle will of course tend to see what may issue from a renewed reflection upon received knowledge or on the foundations for the practice they pursue as quite inconsequential. It is these analysts that Roazen designates as naive—"people regularly talking about Freud's 'discoveries,' instead of more modestly accepting the idea that in actuality what he was doing was forwarding a special way of looking at things" (1992:7).

In the previous chapter the divided attitude of psychoanalysis with regard to its own knowledge was touched upon, together with its desire to take knowledge as a given and a guideline for analytical practice, but still without leaving necessary room for creative theoretical work. At least to some extent this may be assigned to the (unholy) alliance arising between an excluding group—the training analysts—and those excluded, together with the paradoxical sense of shared values that this informal social system gives rise to. To codify what in fact it is that one gathers around, some kind of institutional authority is established, most often around a certain theory or theoretician:

> Groups share ideals of treatment and process. These ideals are embedded in shared fantasies carrying superego value and power. When analysts struggle with regressive factors in the judgement of reality, knowledge and belief must be supported by authorities who are taken as externalised representatives of superego authority. . . . The application of theory at any level of clinical work offers the possibility of a covert or unconscious appeal to authority. [Grossman 1995:889–890]

Thus develops the social foundation for a complex of more or less institutionalized attitudes and views. Such a complex might possibly be designated with what I call *the arrogance of Knowledge*. By this I mean a not uncommon result that comes about when we allow ourselves to be seduced by Knowledge's implicit promise of power, tempting us to believe that we may be in possession of superior insights.[27]

Presumably because he had the opportunity to observe this

very tendency, at the end of his life Freud explicitly warned against the risk that psychoanalysis should develop into a *Weltanschauung*, something he describes as "an intellectual construction which solves all the problems of our existence uniformly on the basis of one overriding hypothesis, which, accordingly, leaves no question unanswered and in which everything that interests us finds its fixed place" (Freud 1933:158).[28] Despite the warning, knowing's transformation into a view of reality is a recurrent phenomenon that seems to haunt the psychoanalytic project, and in fact "Freud's statement that psychoanalysis must not be a *Weltanschauung* has served as a pretext for not examining the extent to which it actually functions as one" (Figueira, as apostrophized in Bernardi and Nieto 1992:142).

In Kernberg's terms for a fictitious analytical ruler it is emphasized that "the main objective of psychoanalytic education is not to help students to acquire what is known in order to develop new knowledge, but to acquire well-proven knowledge regarding psychoanalysis to avoid its dilution, distortion, deterioration and misuse" (1996:1039). A classic example of psychoanalysis as a *Weltanschauung* is the analyst's relation to Freud and his work: "To challenge Freud's theories has usually been responded to with anxiety, as if a sacrilegious outrage were being perpetuated" (Sutherland 1980:842). Arlow describes how his attempt to reduce the study of Freud at an institute fell on deaf ears (1982:14), and Ellman tells us how Winnicott was received with a totally hostile attitude at a reading of a paper at the New York Psychoanalytic Society in 1968 (1996:91), presumably for the reason that he presented ideas that were not "kosher" according to the then prevailing order.

Reed conducted a detailed investigation of how one of the central conceptions of American ego psychology—the transference neurosis—not only guides the analyst's conception of what constitutes clinical facts, but also establishes a divide in his perception between what he actually is taking part in and what (the idealized) theory wants him to apprehend. Thus develops a double registration of experience: "What people do clinically and what they think they ought to do according to the codified rules of technique are not always the same" (Reed 1994:19). One of Reed's respondents says: "If someone asks you, under formal circumstances, what you mean by a transference neurosis, what you respond often depends on the local political situation. [. . . The use of the term] soon became a way of distinguishing between true believers and nonbelievers, between those who were good analysts and those who weren't good analysts" (Reed 1994:57–58).

Grotstein describes how a serious problem cropped up after the APA had decreed that the Los Angeles Institute must rid itself of its Kleinians or else be excluded from the association: "It had not really dawned on me until that moment that I could lose my status as a training analyst because I used such words as 'splitting' and 'projective identification' rather than 'repression' and the 'Oedipus complex'" (1985:39). In an interview conducted by Nosek and Lemlij (1997), past president of the IPA, Leo Rangell, says:

> There is a great deal to say about the massive proliferation of theories in the modern era. While there are many defenders of this trend, and some valid reasons to see this as an increase in creativity, I would have us not lose sight of the losses incurred when established and verified gains are derailed frivolously, or for affective reasons, making for splintering and fragmentation rather than unification and coherence of knowledge. One of the goals of theory is completeness with parsimony. The original elegance and beauty of psychoanalytic theory, when it first captured the imagination, was its promise to explain the most by the least. In no way did this preclude continuous growth and development of the central, expanding body of knowledge. Today, a hundred years later, what I think we have is the danger of destruction or at least erosion of the unique psychoanalytic method of study and treatment, and the theory of understanding of human behavior which meant so much when it appeared on the intellectual scene 100 years ago. To me this plays as central a part as external factors in the disillusionment of the public with our science and discipline.[29]

For anyone existing within such a context the striving to arrive at one's own stand must be accompanied by the fear of challenging authority (or its representatives). That fear, in turn, is presumably connected with the danger of getting caught in the firing line of the chosen authority's hate. Here it is inconsequential whether we are dealing with manifest hate or with a hate projected in fantasy from one's superego reservoir onto the authority. Kernberg seems to lean toward the former:

> Strengthen the graduation rituals by whatever intelligent means you find: this is a field with great potentialities. For example, you may ask the candidates to write up a case for graduation, and then subject their manuscripts to numerous revisions and corrections. Through this experience the candidates acquire a healthy respect for the enormous difficulties in writing an acceptable paper for publication. Or else, require the candidate to present a paper before the psychoanalytic society. The discussants should be the most senior members of that society (who may not have written a paper themselves for a long time). Their demanding expectations of what a scientific paper should include may be communicated by the exhaustive criticism of the candidate's presentation. [1996:1033]

When the arrogance of Knowledge is put in the service of fear, paranoia, and hostility, it easily develops into a mania for perceiving something pathological, aberrant, and immature everywhere, a penchant for always finding fault, which so often permeates collegial relations (even though one does make an effort not to let it show).

In any case, the end result is that all too many find "good reason" to subordinate themselves to the demands of authority and not present their views to their colleagues—and, what is even worse, abstain from thinking altogether: "Presenting ideas to a psychoanalytic audience involves a special risk. This audience is primarily interested in the underlying workings of the personality. To expose internal processes of the writer is to risk uninvited analytic suppositions about one's own personality" (Morrison and Evaldson 1990:414).

It is not uncommon to stumble in the literature upon comments like "[theoretical] divergence should be examined extremely carefully since it may be being used primarily in the service of rationalising personal disturbances" (Schafer 1994:360), and Rangell writes that the theory elected to replace an accepted one is comparable to a symptom (1982:38). Schafer is not necessarily wrong, but his way of making his point cannot but give support to the general conservative interests of the psychoanalytical superego and to the will to stigmatize that is born out of externalized hate. On the whole, traces of such thinking often crop up in the kind of internal criticism that Rangell exemplifies above, deploring in more or less harsh fashion the existence of all these "theoreticians" who are more interested in coining new concepts than expanding established knowledge.[30] Still, the greater danger here is not the humiliation of mental divestiture or no longer being appreciated, but in no longer being allowed to belong. Thus for example, as Britton writes, the anxiety in publishing—that is to say, taking part in theoretical work—"emanates from a fear of criticism by third parties who are regarded as authoritative and *fear of disaffiliation* from colleagues with whom the author feels the need to be *affiliated*" (1997:14, italics in original).[31]

> What is told about clinical technique often has the character of fiction. It shows in the split between what analysts really do and what they say they do.
> —J. Cremerius 1987:1082

> The privacy of our work engenders a pervasive anxiety about whether it conforms to the psychoanalytic canon. Any clinical presentation made by one practitioner to another always, in some form or another, carries the need to reaffirm one's membership and one's right to be a member of the psychoanalytic community. Each time a clinical presentation is made and the participants survive, the ghost of the wild analyst can once again, at least for the time being, be laid to rest.
> —L. Spurling 1997:68

It is an internationally known fact that among active psycho-analysts only a fraction choose to articulate their experience in the form of goal-directed theoretical work. It would seem as if most of those contributing to the theoretical discussion are already on safe ground, which is to say that they are training analysts (see King 1989:344). The majority of those quoted in this investigation are training analysts (and among them, most are men).[32]

> I have been impressed and depressed by the observation that applicants for training often seem to be more creative than the psychoanalysts who graduate from our training institutes. Perhaps our method for selecting candidates is faulty, but in all candour, we must also face the possibility that our training programmes and the atmosphere of our institutes may stultify the creative imagination of our students. [Greenson 1969:504; see also Kernberg 1986:806]

John Gedo, prominent editor and writer in American psychoanalysis, writes that publication is sparse among psychoanalysts, and the common restraint on the literature published is that contributions from schools other than one's own are rejected and that our ideals of equality have lowered demands to such a degree that "at least half of the published analytic literature is devoid of merit" (1996:4). I believe this phenomenon may very well be attributed to a tendency to move only within the wake of some established theoretical authority, which is so common among writers of analytical publications (see Langs 1978:202–203).

> It is my impression, shared with those who have considered this area, that a major factor in the decline of psychoanalysis as a respected body of scientific understanding and as treatment modality, is based, in part, on the failure of analysts, individually and collectively, to sustain the necessary disequilibria and mastery required for the slow incorporation of original ideas into its main body of knowledge and technical functioning. [Langs 1978:198; see also Stone 1975:343–345][33]

The reality evoked by quotations like the ones above is not uniformly dark. As has been said, psychoanalysis has existed in a state of constant evolution and change since its inception, not least when it comes to the last twenty-five years or so, when discussions have been quite lively and variegated. Despite the low number of analysts publishing, so many articles and books are produced that no analyst can fully follow all that is being offered for discussion.

During the third epoch of the psychoanalytic institution, those voices raised demanding censorship and allegiance have not been the only ones heard; there have always been others advocating theoretical plurality and development. We have already acquainted ourselves with Balint's critique of the system. In 1951 Rickman writes that "creative imagination, no matter how inconvenient to our complacency, must be given the fullest scope" (p. 223). A quarter of a century later Stone says: "I am less concerned about the stormy irrationalities of militant dissidence than the prevailing rigidity in my own intellectual community" (1975:345). From Dorn: "A psychoanalytic society should be a place where new ideas are welcomed. . . . To the extent that new ideas are not welcome, we lack the potential to encourage creativity. . . . The analytic society is the place to present new ideas and 'research' in progress" (1982–1983:699). Kernberg, who in later years has been one of the most astute critics of the prevailing (third epoch) system writes in 1993: "I see the proliferation of alternative theoretical models—the British object relations, self psychology, the hermeneutic approach, interpersonal analysis, the Lacanian school—less as a threat and more as a spur to psychoanalytic development, a potential enriching of theory and technique, and as a stimulus to research" (p. 48).

But the true problem has never been a lack of critical voices or of open-minded analysts; the problem is that "the organizational distortions in psychoanalytic institutes are self-perpetuating" (Kernberg 1986:826). The critical voices keep repeating approximately the same things because the basis of the problems addressed—which, according to the interpretation of reality proffered here, is the superego complex—never seems to be affected by prevalent critique. Therefore on the societal level, in many respects, and too often, there is a substantial lack of exploratory dialogue:

> It is guaranteed that all psychoanalysts writing for their "colleagues" today will encounter, at least among some readers, disbelief at their failure to grasp basic principles, headshaking over their hubris in imagining that what they have written contains new ideas, or disinterest from readers not of their "school" because they talk "another language" that is too "old fashioned" or "not really psychoanalysis." [Elliott and Spezzano 2000a:15]

Groups and societies may differ, but can avoid serious discussion by staying away from any heated issues and keeping all relations "cool"; societies may choose to keep everything totally silent when it comes to contributions coming from "dissidents" within one's own group or any other one. At the same time, total freedom may be given to all: "So far . . . organized psychoanalysis survived a number of modifications but has not yet developed a productive technique of communicating among different modifiers. The next generation of psychoanalysts will have to find ways to subject the modification to rational procedure so that their contributions can be tested against each other" (Bergmann 1993:950–951)

THE PSYCHOANALYST'S INNER CAREER

Prescription and Ethos

In our theoretical exposition above, it was claimed that the professional superego is both a prescriptive and a proscriptive factor internalized by anyone accepted as a member of a professional body, forming a tie securely uniting the members of the group. Just like the analyst's dependency upon his organization rests upon valid professional needs, the superego is also a carrier of positive professional functions. These are the prescriptive ones, specifying what the professional should know in theory and in practice, what his relations with clients and the representatives of other professions should look like, and so forth. In this sense the superego may be said to support a professional *ethos* and as such it must surely be an indispensable aspect of any professional identity.[34]

Within the scope of the professional superego we find not only its conscious and unconscious injunctions, but everything from codifications such as by-laws of psychoanalytic societies, the rules and procedures for training institutes, the technical precepts of the practice itself, and a written set of professional ethical rules to the *primum est non nocere* of the Hippocratic oath[35] and the responsibility to be a keeper in the service of the analytical setting and the conscience of the analysis (Calef and Weinshel 1980:283). In this way the individual analyst amasses a set of rules and precepts specifying which kinds of actions are correct and which are erroneous. The prescriptive aspect of the superego keeps watch over the moral dimension of the profession.[36]

For psychoanalysis, the importance of this moral dimension for its survival as a unitary discipline cannot be overestimated. Analytical praxis is an activity and a concomitant experience which, despite the fact of its dispersal in relatively small groups all across the world and despite at times rather harsh differences in theory, can show such a uniformity in its practical application that most analysts testify that on the clinical level more often than not they will understand each other's work.

I have devoted relatively little attention to this prescriptive aspect because it is not as connected to an immanent pedagogy as the proscriptive aspect and does not have the same inhibiting effects. Even though it is of marginal interest for our immediate concerns it is still important as an element in the psychoanalyst's professional development.

Some commentators will perceive only the prescriptive aspect of the superego. Such is the case with Fliess, for example, who, when speaking of the analytical superego and its relation to the analytical work ego writes that "the superego's judicial function becomes . . . what might be called the analyst's 'therapeutic conscience' and its function of critical self-observation enables the analyst's ego to achieve that singular detachment towards its own psychic content, conscious as well as preconscious, which we found so indispensable for his work" (1942:222; see also Blum 1981:552–553).

Initially, the superego may be felt as a support and a relief, but it is important to note that as the moral dimension is tied to the injunctions coming from a superego, hate will lurk somewhere in the background. As long as the analyst's functions are carried out as a response to these precepts, they will operate in an atmosphere of fear. The subject may, of course, be so identified with the dogma that it no longer experiences the voice of the superego as an alien and hostile invasion. But we may recall how Freud characterized the superego as having a "compulsive character which manifests itself in the form of a categorical imperative" (Freud 1923b:35) and for that reason analytical morals will tend to leave traces in the form of a degree of rigidity. Even when, for example, the superego admonishes us to "honor thy father and thy mother," the severity of the demand—not the message itself, be it noted!—is carried by the same hate, even though its more brutal facets may lie hidden or dormant for the moment.

Therefore, even the prescriptive aspect of the professional superego may at times show itself in rather harsh ways, as, for example, in how the body of psychoanalysts as a whole seems to have adopted a working moral borrowed from the medical profession in the service of professional interest. As we have seen, in some countries physicians dominate the profession almost totally. The successful professionalization process of the medical corps at the end of the nineteenth century and the following decades allowed their sense of group loyalty and professional identity to develop to a high degree, with an acute sensitivity to what behooves a practitioner and how he should comport himself. Bourdieu compares the physician to an army leader (1984:90), expected to appear as a hero. The competence demanded of the doctor is primarily of a practical kind; he should have a trustworthy diagnostic gaze, he must be able to deal with critical situations involving questions of life and death with indisputable authority, he must be the leader of a team and be prepared to make great sacrifices for his calling. In Sweden, it has been expected of doctors to work for years on end sixty or seventy hours per week if one includes being on call.[37]

It might be expected that a physician who has chosen to become a psychoanalyst may have distanced himself from at least part of the ethos supporting a readiness for such sacrifices which, even if they are not exactly self-destructive, at least must involve considerable limitations, not least when it comes to family life. But if we consider that there are psychoanalysts who meet analysands from 6:30 in the morning until seven or eight in the evening five days a week, and on top of that are available on the phone from 6:10 until 6:25 before seeing their first patient of the day, it is evident that the heroic ethos of the medical profession has not wholly rubbed off—or at least not from everyone. There are not many voices that can be heard to warn of these tendencies; I have encountered only one:

> Only the highly exceptional individual at the height of his powers can use eleven to twelve hours of psychoanalytic work creatively. Even if we discard a more or less continuous invasion of the psychoanalytic instrument by life circumstances, these work loads tend to create an inner reservation of psychic expenditure which influences the entire day's work. New ideas stimulated by patient material have a fleeting quality, appear on the periphery of consciousness, and may require time for reflection to get hold of them. Psychoanalysts at any age should carefully examine their true working capacity, considering not only their therapeutic effectiveness but their creative potential under changing circumstances. [Bak 1970:19][38]

For lay analysts of varying backgrounds the encounter with the medical heroic ethos is in many ways an encounter with a totally alien tradition. For example, psychologists have always allowed themselves to be much more easygoing than doctors. Medicine is "a practical science whose truth and success matters to the whole nation" (Bourdieu 1984:96), whereas the practice of the psychologist is more seldom a question of life and death. His activities are often of a greater theoretical than practical interest and therefore do not matter to "the whole nation" in the same way. To society, psychology is simply more dispensable than medicine, which makes psychologists grapple with totally different issues when it comes to their professional identity.

For the professional superego of psychoanalysts who are psychologists, the demands originating from the model of some of their physician colleagues have been a strong injection. With the possibility of attaining the rank of psychoanalyst and—something that for several generations has been a unique opportunity for a psychologist (I am not talking only about the United States here)— within this restricted area of competence be regarded on equal footing with the doctors, psychologists have subjected themselves to the heroic ethic without protest, which has been evidenced by how willingly they have submitted to the discipline required of a candidate in analytic training (see the beginning of Chapter 4). In this way, through the immanent pedagogy of its mere form, training results in the internalization of the heroic ethos belonging to the medical profession into the superego.[39]

Decisive Years

I believe that it took me a good ten years of full-time psychoanalytic practice to feel myself a psychoanalyst and be able to accept patients without some degree of guilt and anxiety; and I know that I am not alone in this. The newly qualified analyst is, therefore, confronted with something which might be described as an ego loss. [Klauber 1983:46]

No education is completed just because one has submitted one's apprentice's examination work and received a diploma: "Graduation is only a marker in the training of an analyst, albeit an important one, rather than the point of completion" (Glick et al. 1996:809).

There remains the long road toward finding a personal identity as a psychoanalyst. It is a matter of course that to advance to the rank of Master takes years of serious work, where knowledge is gradually transformed into competence. The time span suggested by Klauber—ten years—is not uncommon in the literature when one wants to indicate how many years this might take.[40] These first long years of independent work seem to be a critical period when the maturing analyst decides how he is going to find a way to handle his superego and develop his own voice as a clinician.

One of the great difficulties involved in "surviving" the first years as an independent analyst/psychotherapist lies in the fact that "we have to make such an extensive commitment to the profession before we have had much opportunity to practice it and develop confidence based on experience" (Buechler 1988:466). How, then, to maintain an acceptable level of professional self-esteem when at the same time one knows and feels that one in some very critical respects is still deficient?

> When people deliver themselves trustingly into our hands as their therapists, unless they know a considerable amount about psychotherapy, which many of them do not, this means exactly what it says: they put their faith in *us*, as people. It is only experience which enables us to feel their faith is justified. At the beginning of a career as therapist, faith in ourselves will of necessity only stem from trusting our wish and intention to do well by these people and to become good therapists; all we have is our awareness of a vocational sense, a strong motivation, and the experience of our own therapy—including an identification with the self-confidence of our own analyst or therapist—on which to rely. When faced with our patients, aware of our inexperience and ignorance, a quantum of anxiety is realistic. It is then that a parallel faith in the therapeutic process we have been trained to use holds us, and evolves quite rapidly with practice—probably more rapidly at first than our faith in ourselves. Until we begin to trust our slowly growing skills, faith in ourselves is tenuous, and sustained largely by patience and hope. Finally, perhaps ten years on from qualification, we re-

alize that faith in the therapeutic process has kept us going until faith in ourselves has drawn level; then the two blend, as anxiety fades and unself-conscious relaxation becomes the keynote of our daily work. [Coltart 1993:107–108, italics in original]

It should not be difficult to appreciate how the first years of an analyst's career are not only difficult, but also perilous, considering the inevitable conflict arising between his capacity to gradually gain self-reliance while at the same time bearing all his insecurities, and his more or less prevalent tendency to seek guidance from his faith in a certain clinical procedure, a certain theory, or identification with the real or in fantasy perfect (training) analyst. In other words, the lurking danger resides—as so very often, it might be added—within the sphere of possible idealizations and a dependency upon "perfection," which quite flexibly will conjoin with the professional superego (see King 1989). "I wonder if, in our fear of changing 'the spirit of analysis,' we too are not apt to respect certain rules so literally that they are transformed into taboos" (Nacht 1962:208).[41]

> In analysis, [the young analyst] has been taught, the pathogenic conflicts are reexperienced in a regressive transference neurosis; interpretations are made within the transference; the material is worked through; the conflicts are resolved; and there results a structural alteration of the personality, a radical character change. So exact is this account that it might have been carved in stone. Nothing of such precision and finality occurs in his consulting room. With his interpretations he writes in water. His patients get better and get worse. Most of them derive some benefit from his efforts, but of structural alterations and radical character changes he sees little. He is forced reluctantly toward the conclusion that psycho-analysis is not what it is represented to be, and he begins to be troubled by a vague sense of fraudulence.
>
> This is a crucial time in his professional life. [Wheelis 1956:179][42]

Summing up his experience as a psychoanalyst at mid-career, Gedo

writes in 1979: "By far the greatest proportion of my analytic failures occurred immediately after my graduation from a psychoanalytic institute, i.e., among the first patients I tried to treat
without supervision" (p. 647).[43] There may be a kernel of truth
in a statement such as "the dissatisfactions and the disappoint-
ments constitute a not insignificant element in the professional
lives of many analysts" (Calef and Weinshel 1980:280), but it is
quite obvious that during these first years there is an impending
risk that the analyst could lose his faith, not only in his own capacities but also in psychoanalysis as such. Such experiences may
turn out to be quite burdensome and "many analysts experience,
in the first decade of their work, strong guilt feelings for not knowing enough" (Bergmann 1997:81). "The guilt and lowered self-
esteem about therapeutic failure might be less if we prepared our
students more adequately for the limitations of psychoanalytic
therapy. In their self-reproaches they look at the picture of Freud
in their office, or think of Phyllis Greenacre, saying to themselves:
'What's wrong with me? They would have succeeded'" (Bak
1970:12). Limentani speaks in this connection of what he calls *post-
graduate breakdown* (1974:76), and Klauber speaks of "the depressive position of the newly qualified analyst" (1986:206).[44]

Wheelis enumerates three paths of development that he sees
as possible responses to these difficulties: (1) retreat to the dogma;
(2) keeping an open mind with critical evaluation of both the theories and one's own clinical experience, despite the increase of inner
conflict that this may entail; (3) the risk of losing faith in the psychoanalytic project, with the concomitant desire to do something
else (1956:179–180). The first kind of response interests us here
because it touches upon the superego complex, as does the second kind of response; a deeper understanding of how it may come
about could give us some clues to how the superego complex may
be counteracted.

The third kind of response is a potential threat to psychoanalysis. The pleasure and satisfaction, which at best can come from
taking part in the praxis of psychoanalysis, are indispensable factors in the analyst's life: "The daily work of therapeutic psycho-

analysis is difficult and often painful for the analyst. He needs a certain amount of positive pleasure in the performance of his duties to enable him to sustain a lively interest in and concern for the goings-on in his patients" (Greenson 1966:21). If that joy is lacking he will in one way or another abandon or fail the task for which he has sacrificed so much. The risk implied is not only that psychoanalysis could lose adherents, but that it could produce renegades who in their disappointment threaten to become its sworn enemies. A milder form of this reaction might be a chronic lack of meaningfulness in work, something which, of course, will have an adverse affect on analysands.[45]

I suggest that the way psychoanalytic training is organized can be unconsciously responded to by some psychoanalysts whose false self "adapts and alters itself in response to forced environmental pressures," as an experience that alienates them from their true selves and their own identity, though they do retain some of this "not-me" quality of the compliance, and hence a deep feeling of dissatisfaction (King 1989:339).

With the crisis that the young analyst has to go through, and at the threshold of either one of the three possibilities mentioned by Wheelis, he is faced with some kind of ethical decision where his integrity is at stake: "Resentment and negative feelings left unexpressed are indicative not only of the lack of courage of conviction, but a 'passive dishonesty,' thereby allowing something to continue, constituting in effect a co-conspiracy with what one, in all good conscience, disapproves—a form of betrayal of an ego-ideal" (Aarons 1982–1983:686).[46]

Fogel and Glick write that within "good" institutes and societies one creates the means for collegial support to facilitate the working through of these critical states, with the important addendum that the *personal and institutional resistances* (against acknowledging the problems at hand) may be formidable and that the wished-for processes of working through are not to be taken for granted (1991:417).[47] Considering the superego complex's seemingly permanent presence in the interaction between analysts and their institutions, one may surmise that resistances against owning

206 HATE AND LOVE IN PSYCHOANALYTICAL INSTITUTIONS

up to the difficulties are quite substantial, and that therefore the institutional forms for the working through of those problems may be seriously neglected.

One important factor behind this resistance is that the superego —despite all the misery it may give rise to—easily becomes something the subject will not gladly part with (not unlike how it may relate to a symptom). In its capacity as an internalized parental authority the superego becomes a cherished possession "with the help of [which] the ego 'participates' in the more powerful father's might, and the acquisition of the superego is the equivalent of the acquisition of a trophy" (Fenichel quoted in Szasz 1958:605).[48] The trophy will be especially valuable to the subject when it is transformed in that operation we met with above under the rubric "identification with the aggressor." In such instances power and glory may seem to be the subject's unswerving allies.

When the idealizations of the method, the theory, and the perfect analyst combine with the love for the professional superego it is easy for the analyst to get stuck with attitudes that will finally make him a suitable instrument of the institutional superego system.[49] Concerning just which attitudes these may be there are probably as many suggestions as there are commentators. I make no claim to cover this area, but restrict myself to some simple reflections.

Orthos Doxa

Giovacchini describes how analysts at the beginning of their career often are "more catholic than the Pope" (1985:7) and how psychoanalytic ideals of purity could make personal feelings, anxieties, or needs stand out as utterly blasphemous. Indeed a telling image of the unholy alliance between idealizations and loyalty to the superego may issue not only in strict self-control, but via identification with the aggressor in a tendency to control the environment. This is one possible way of accounting for the phenomenon often referred to as its orthodoxy. *Orthos doxa*—the correct doctrine—is an intellectual instrument to keep oneself and others in check so that everything stays in accordance with the structure and the rule which, by dint of the immanent pedagogy, has become part of the professional superego.

On the level of clinical experience this will result in strict superego demands: "Analysts often act as though they feel that, within themselves, they should know what it is necessary to say or to talk about at every moment" (Schafer 1997a:170). Not least is he expected to know what, according to the theoretical canon of his chosen system of knowledge, is stirring within the analysand and how he should formulate his interventions. Slavin (1992) describes how candidates embarking upon their first supervised cases reject and criticize their own previous therapeutic skillfulness and that of others, instead maintaining an idealized conception of how "truly analytical" interventions should be presented.[50] That such reactions should exist only among candidates seems improbable—they are surely common with newly graduated analysts also.

Knowledge is indispensable for any discipline, but such an insight must not be allowed to fog the fact that orthodoxy's strict demands for knowledge run the risk of producing technical rigidity and a way of relating to the analysand that is both unimaginative and unnecessarily impersonal. Steltzer writes in this connection of an "instrumental dissociation" arising when the analyst manages to split himself so that one part is feeling, while the other observes the feeling part:

> We are trained to function like that to achieve understanding, and that form of mental functioning becomes the principle to which we adjust our everyday practice as clinicians. If working conditions have something to do with identity formation, one result of this kind of training would be the deformation of the candidate's identity. . . . Even if it is not obvious, it appears that candidates . . . enter training in order to be taught how to be less sensitive to the other's unconscious. What they get is a way of working, a way of relating to their patients' unconscious

which, though uncomfortable, is less painful than feeling the dreams and nightmares of their patients. The pay-off is the transformation of the sensitive candidate into a schizoid-alexithymic (split and unable to dream) professional. [Steltzer 1986:71–73]

Despite all discussion taking place during the last twenty-five years or so concerning the processual character of analytic understanding, its hermeneutic character, and its inherent contextuality, the notions of "correct understanding" and the "correct interpretation" live on with stubborn, not to say persecutory, perseverance in the private ideational world of many analysts. Wallerstein speaks of "our conflict- and anxiety-based reluctance to recognize clearly the true (and modest) limits of our knowledge" and "the wide discrepancy . . . between what we feel that our theory requires of us that we should know and what we realistically do know" (1981a:290).

The Tyranny of Interpretations

Despite differing ways of conceptualizing the matter, there is great agreement among analysts that interpretation—what I spoke of as "interpreting" in Chapter 2—is perhaps the most central line of communication from analyst to analysand. A noninterpretive psychoanalysis would be an oxymoron. But interpretation can, as we have seen, easily become part of the kind of mutual power games in which people so readily indulge.

The superego says: "The principal responsibility of the future analyst . . . is to make the correct interpretation" (Arlow 1982:17). When interpretation has assumed this position within the analyst's ideational world there is something fearsome on its way, for interpretation is in no way the simple expression of love—I would rather say that interpretation actually grows from a sublimated form of hate.

Now, how would that figure?

Hate has been mentioned as a basic form for the subject's way of relating to its world, primarily as it precipitates in the form of an impulse to extinguish whatever is foreign, in particular the Other. As such, hate will, of course, be a serious threat to life within any culture and that is why man has learned to domesticate its force by sublimation to the degree that it can even operate "in the service of the ego." In a first step, the blind impulse to annihilate is sublimated into a striving to take possession of the Other and reduce him to the status of slave. In this way, hate as a purely destructive force is transformed into the subject's impulse to make itself master of all that it can encompass within its very own categories, be it the Other himself or his property. The intersubjective play vacillating between the dominance of one and the submission of the Other, which in this way will arise, is only partly acceptable to any form of civilized intercourse. Therefore, the raw appropriation of the Other implied in setting oneself up as his master must undergo yet another process of refinement, whereby impulses to either annihilate or subdue the Other are transformed—in the service of the ego—into the will to interpret. The fact that all interpretation bears a legacy taken from the violent potential of hate shows in how interpretation assimilates and subjugates what is truly unfamiliar in the Other into something digestible, into the stuff proper to the ego, or, what is perhaps even worse, into the categories of theory.

The newly graduated psychoanalyst's difficulty in interpreting is often the result of theory not having been assimilated: "I tried too hard to understand my patients theoretically. Sometimes, at least according to theory as I understood it, my patients seemed to have two left feet, or two right; the theoretical shoes fit poorly, but I forced them on anyhow" (Spruiell 1984:26). One great obstacle to the assimilation of theory is that it may have become so idealized that it would seem a crime to deconstruct it. When theory under such conditions comes to be used in the clinical situation it becomes a model for interpretation, something that does support good analytic work, but deters the analyst from listening to his own presence together with the analysand.[51]

A basic factor—a basic terror, one might say—in the development of the analyst's professional superego is the fact that the analyst has been interpreted in his own analysis. Interpretation is probably one of, if not *the* major factor in the training analysis conducive to the kind of normalization of the candidate discussed in the previous chapter. When the hate he thus has suffered comes to be introjected, it can return in the form of a demand from the superego that he should now himself interpret. Precisely through that action hate can revert back to the external world and once again partake in the grand circulation.

However indispensable it may be for the analytic project, interpretation is a double-edged sword that must be handled with humility. That so many authors have felt the need to point this out must have to do with the very tangible risk that the analyst, in spite of all, might fail to grasp the seriousness of the matter.

The Hermeneutics of Suspicion

In his monumental study, *Freud and Philosophy*, Paul Ricoeur (1965) coined the expression "hermeneutics of suspicion" to designate the code that with Marx, Nietzsche, and Freud became part of modern self-reflection and that insists with its message that there is always a hidden meaning to be excavated from beneath our manifest expressions. The benevolent understanding of this is that the hermeneutics of suspicion is tantamount to the realization that knowledge and self-understanding are relative and that they can always be criticized, reevaluated, and reformulated. In its "tougher" version, the hermeneutics of suspicion becomes a tool for the ego's will to power and a support for the general human tendency to want to rule over one's fellow man whenever possible. Within the psychoanalytic context this will result in the (most dubitable) claim that "What you are saying in fact means something else than what you think it does—and I am the one who *knows*." One must not underestimate the omnipotent satisfaction that can be experienced by anyone believing himself capable of mastering the unconscious.

Suspicion, along with its promise of power, tempts the analyst to adjust himself to a world in which he presumes himself to be in possession of superior knowledge of human desires and motives. The notion that there is a correct doctrine and a correct exposition of it makes the concepts involved lose their heuristic capacity, and they transform into doctrinary elements in a system of thinking that has succumbed to the arrogance of Knowledge. Thus is established a *Weltanschauung* which, to be sure, develops a fundamental distrust and an equally deplorable tendency in the psychoanalyst to find fault with everything, not only in relation to his own colleagues, but in the world at large. Not only candidate selection, but collegial discourse in general will then become "a clinical conference in advanced psychopathology" of the kind that Eisendorfer spoke of (1959:374).

By dint of such convictions, acquired to serve as a defense against the inherent uncertainties of the profession, it then turns out that "analysts often (always?) think they know what is going on in a patient's mind better than the patient does" (Brenner 1996:23). If it were so simple that the whole matter would limit itself to orthodoxy lending itself to the ego's will to power, things might not be all that bad. What is worse is that the hermeneutics of suspicion becomes a cunning way of satisfying the professional superego's demand for *orthos doxa* while at the same time avoiding being oneself the target of any suspicion. If the analyst is the one who *knows*, the analysand is, by definition, the one who is both unsophisticated and ignorant.[52] The analyst's identification with the aggressor allows him then to let the analysand carry the potential guilt and/or shame for not "doing right" and not being in the know.

The psychoanalytic conception of transference is necessary for the understanding of the analytical process so that it may be handled in its "intended way." But it is hardly controversial to claim that this notion of a force within the analysand making him apt to project all kinds of qualities and feelings onto the analyst is also a potential instrument of power to the latter. In the name of transference it is possible to deny or obfuscate the input of the analyst's own qualities, idiosyncrasies, or mistakes, and instead maintain that it is all a question of the analysand's distorted perceptions. It must be acknowledged that quite a number of more or less traumatizing excesses have been perpetrated in this fashion and that they surely have satisfied a claim for power.

> Not only have analysts tended to deny, and failed to appreciate, the patient's unconscious therapeutic efforts on their behalf, but individually and collectively, they have tended to be almost totally absorbed with the patient's pathological, transference-based functioning and his destructive intentions vis-à-vis the analytic experience and the analyst—this, to the virtual exclusion of the patient's valid, nontransference-based functioning and his creative endeavors within the analytic situation. The patient as enemy, his creativity to be envied and destroyed, has insidiously dominated the psychoanalyst's view of his analysand. Relatively few analysts have acknowledged and attempted to comprehend the analysand's extensive positive functioning and potential within the analytic relationship. [Langs 1978:200; see also Marmor 1953][53]

Thus, in collegial discussions one may sometimes apprehend a kind of pleasurable triumph coming to the fore as some analysts "unmask" their own analysands or those of their colleagues, displaying the "true" or "deeper" meanings of the unconscious fantasies supporting their "resistance," determining their "unanalyzability," or proving their "destructiveness."[54] Suspicion may easily turn into a superego terror coming from analysts who, for example, "are united in deifying the belief that putting preverbal fantasies into words gives them the very omnipotent control they seem constantly to find in their patients" (Greenson 1969:511; see also Wallerstein 1981a:289).

At institutions where the hermeneutics of suspicion is vigorous, there is an obvious risk that it will contribute to the alienation of potential and even present analysands from the psychoanalytic experience, thus furthering the loss of patients taking place in so many countries today.

From Superego to Ego Ideal

By now that voice of my own superego has been tamed
to a softer tone of an ego-ideal. The message that voice
speaks is now more of values than of threat.
                                        —W. Poland 1985:149[55]

The psychoanalyst's *inner career*[56] stands in contrast to the external career attainable in most other professions, where one's work and actions are more or less on public display, making it possible to receive the attention and appreciation (and sometimes criticism) of the surroundings, and perhaps even win fame. Such dimensions are not altogether absent in the professional life of the psychoanalyst, but that part of his career that has to do with the praxis closest to him is, on the whole, closed off from view. Being inner and private—and therefore lacking much of the support that would have been provided by an audience, collegial or other-wise—the analyst's career relies upon an inner process of solitary self-reflection, perhaps more so than in other vocations.

In this sense, the analyst's inner career has to do with an ethi-cal dimension that is a question rather of "values than of threat," where the analyst gradually reflects upon his task and how he may have been successful or failed at meeting the demands of its "in-tended ways." This evidently has to do with a dimension of the analyst's professional development which, at least potentially, may stand apart from its moral dimension as it usually is codified, say, for example, in the common rules of the trade that we previ-ously associated with the prescriptive and positive aspects of the professional superego.

It seems that only few have sought to describe or make theory of the psychoanalyst's inner career. To some extent this state of things may be ascribed to the fact that the analytic experience itself is such a fragile one and not easily shared—psychoanalysis is certainly a private affair for both parties of the dyad. It may also have to do with a lack of institutions for tracking and/or assisting such processes. Then again, it might be an issue relating to the professional superego: "Perhaps because as psychoanalysts we have been busy with what we thought we were supposed to be like, we have given very little thought to how we actually utilize what we are taught and how we change ourselves, our minds, and our ways of practicing" (Reed 1994:15).[57]

To pursue this, let us begin to ask ourselves what kind of "substance" we might consider superego and ego ideal to be composed of. In 1914, while Freud is still working over the concept of an ego ideal he writes that this is something "imposed from without. . . . What prompted the subject to form an ego ideal . . . arose from the critical influence of his parents (*conveyed to him by the medium of the voice*)" (1914a:96, my italics). The same idea recurs in "The Ego and the Id," where he is even more explicit, pointing out that it is "impossible for the superego . . . to disclaim its origin from things heard" (Freud 1923b:52).[58] Following the parents there will be all the voices belonging to the whole row of authorities that appear in the life of someone growing up.

To the repertoire of things having been "conveyed by the medium of the voice," we may also add such things as fragments of what we ourselves and others have said, fractions of narratives and truncated sentences, inflections, and idiosyncratic expressions. The elements within this register I call *narrathemes*.[59] Narrathemes make up a wide-ranging set of words, judgments, and formulations, more or less always ready-at-hand for the subject to utilize in his speaking and narrating reflecting activity, as it interprets and evaluates its life and actions, its desires and affects. Essentially, the analyst's inner career has to do with a gradual displacement—through a process of self-reflection—from the concerns of the emotional sphere of his superego to those of his ego ideal; from hate and the fear and potential feeling of threat that this may engender (and of which we have seen several examples in this chapter), to the emotional economy of the ego ideal, which I would like to designate as libidinous in the sense that it is mainly characterized by such aims as interest (in the Other) and self-esteem. Therefore it also touches upon "more of values than of threat."

In Chapter 2 I suggested that the good belonging to a certain praxis perhaps cannot be defined, but only practiced. This in no way, however, excludes the possibility that the analyst is immersed in a sea of narrathemes designated to give word to the good of psychoanalysis, ranging from the now familiar enumerations of desired characteristics (virtues) to the prescriptions of how concrete clinical situations should be handled. The difficult—if not to say the tragic—matter is that everything appearing within this genre may just as easily lend itself to use in the service of the superego as that of the ego ideal. Thus, what is said may not be what is decisive, the important factor being within what kind of economy it is being transmitted and received. Furthermore, what once may have been transmitted within the economy of the superego can free itself from its intimate connection with hate, so that it may instead enter the libidinous economy of the ego ideal.

How, then, can an introjected narratheme take on the function of an ego ideal? When thought of as a set of narrathemes, the ego ideal should not be construed as a mental representation having the function of a model, but rather as a locus from which are constantly repeated decisive questions concerning the subject's existential position and direction, plus its self-monitoring evaluation of these. Let us say that certain narrathemes in this respect occupy a special place insofar as they are not merely in the service of the general interpreting activities whereby we reflect upon and understand our existence, but rather insistently (and at times irritatingly) they come back to us with a recurring series of issues that in the final count will seem inevitable to us. When narrathemes of that kind enter a libidinous economy our analyst is provided with a thematic structure that ultimately compels him to seek some kind of answer to a mystery of central importance to him: it is this thematic structure that I identify as the ego ideal.

To make this abstract reasoning somewhat more tangible, let us imagine an analyst confronted with Bion's injunction, "Do not remember past sessions" (1967:260), a phrase I will regard as a narratheme for our present use. This is an interesting example because it is quite tempting to take this to be a form of communication from the superego, as Bion actually writes in the following section that his admonishments "must be obeyed *all* the time and not simply during the sessions." In other words, it is easy to hear a "*Thou shalt not* remember past sessions!"

But, to the extent that our analyst manages to withstand the pressure of hate issuing from the superego to some satisfactory degree, he will, owing to the narratheme, repeatedly be brought back to that very formulation that reminds him to ask himself: "What is it that makes a good psychoanalyst?" The return of this notion to our analyst's personal and self-reflective narrative will leave him with no other option than to produce some meaningful and personal answer, which will happen as, for example, he fantasizes and asks himself, "What *is* it, in fact, not to remember past sessions?" "How will sessions be influenced if I still do?" "Will something really different happen when I don't?" Thus is laid the foundation for an ethical dimension in the subject's self-reflection as it evaluates real and fantasized actions against the thematic structure of the ideal.

In relation to the commandments of the superego there is never room enough for the personal narrative to be playfully exploratory, as one of the main objectives of the superego is to decide whether or not the subject deserves condemnation. In contradistinction to that, the questioning attitude of the ego ideal will have a summoning or exhorting quality, as when it is connected with a kernel of self-esteem and then may represent such aims as, for example, are built into all those notions of how the analyst conceptualizes the "good" or the "right" way of carrying out his task—which is to say along its "intended paths." Here we find the foundations for a personal professional ethic, as there can really be no attempt to answer the question, "What is the nature of the task at hand?" which will not simultaneously and in some degree be a reply to queries like "How would I like to be performing it?" or "Wherein lies its good?" This ethical dimension is at the heart of our self-reflective activity and is implied in every attempt of mine to ascertain what it is I am doing. It is not, then, primarily connected with maintaining oneself in relation to a model or an ideal already at hand in the form an explicit and complete notion existing *outside* or *before* my reflection. Instead, the evaluation of actual and possible actions arises all the while as I reflect through my narrative (and perhaps especially when this takes place through the use of these specific narrathemes)—the personal narration of our experience and the story of what good work is all about are parts of one and the same process. Only after the fact is the norm for good work established which, in turn, may be formulated as an ideal and thus become a new narratheme: "The quotidian of doing analysis . . . does not arise from maxims; on the contrary, maxims are principles derived from good clinical work. Such a position comes imperceptibly—as a consequence—with experience, provided there is a deep commitment to the core of our discipline" (Spruiell 1984:28). The ego ideal offers a thematic for the project of personal narrative to establish a conception of self that the subject may rely upon, and in its image it may experience a sense of self-esteem. With this kind of self-love, we do not mean narcissistic preoccupation or entrenchment, but rather a warm and benevolent self-reflection comprising anything ranging from free and desire-driven fantasying to a more austere self-examination where our empirical ego and our actions are judged against the background of the orientation elicited by the ideal.[60]

> There's a lot of love that goes into our work. I think we do everybody a disservice to the extent to which we deny that and minimize it. When I say love, I'm talking about self-love as well. I need my patients every bit as much in my way as they need me. And that's why, at age 73, I'm not reluctant to go on. I'm very reluctant to stop because I get fed by it. And I believe that if we can't acknowledge that, we're just destroying the large part of what we try to do. [James McLaughlin, quoted in Raymond and Rosbrow-Reich 1997:335]

But with these ways of reasoning have we not ended up in a self-confirmatory circle, where the transition from superego to ego ideal presupposes an already established libidinal economy of the latter? Both yes and no. I believe that reflective activity itself is the very precondition for any such transition. Thus we come up against a kind of paradox, where the subject, against all odds, must resist the power of the superego. Only with courage can that space be cleared where the libidinal economy of the ego ideal might be established.

The most important room for reflection is the analyst's every-day—not to say commonplace—personal narrative, with its strident stream of simple whims and fancies together with more complex constructions where he summarizes, interprets, and evaluates his existence while at the same time drawing the contours of a possible future. In analytic circles the more elaborated versions of this have traditionally been called "self-analysis." Thus Joseph writes, for example, that "the capacity to think, feel, and react as a psychoanalyst" requires continued *self-analysis*, studies, and psychoanalytic work (1983:14–15). Whether or not this kind of self-reflection ought to be called "analysis," the fact remains that it is within this activity that the most important work is carried out, for the very simple reason that the personal narrative's reflection upon lived experience is something that the human subject is always immersed in.

The dialogical interpreting of the psychoanalytic situation is probably one of the most sophisticated forms of self-reflection attainable. However, the newly graduated analyst has often just finished with his training analysis and is therefore not only economically weak, but also occupied with the task of acquainting himself with his new occupation. Therefore the dialogue necessary for the transition from superego to ego ideal will perhaps more often take place within the confines of various institutionalized forums for theoretical and clinical discussion, such as conversations or seminars between colleagues, where it becomes necessary to somehow question and reinterpret central aspects of received knowledge.[61]

Another form of reflection comes with supervision. It would be an exception if, during his first years of independent work, the newly graduated analyst were not to seek regular supervision, individually or in collegial groups—in the latter case either together with others in the same phase of professional development, or perhaps more formally with elder members of the society or guest supervisors visiting from other societies.[62] Just as important is the experience of conducting supervision himself. Here the supervising analyst must formulate his views and opinions in a way that will have repercussions in his own work.

And finally: theoretical work. The main points concerning this activity have been presented in Chapter 2. All I wish to add here is that constructive theoretical work is indispensable for the analyst to discover for himself where he actually stands.

The newly graduated analyst's struggle to find his own voice, clinically and theoretically, is a long and hard way to go. Whatever shape this process may take, freedom of thought is necessary for the young analyst to reflect upon and evaluate his personal experience. Therefore it is important to know not only what his previous experience of supervision may have looked like, but also how the institutions surrounding the postgraduate will tend to such issues.

As was seen in the previous chapter, it easily happens that the professional superego precipitates to form informal but still quite robust institutions and attitudes designed to avert colleagues from discarding their conformity with orthodoxy. Even when the psychoanalytical society functions in accordance with its intended ways, as was described at the beginning of this chapter—as a support for analytical values, the analytic attitude, and the analyst as the caretaker of the analytical setting—this function is most often geared to the needs of the elderly or more advanced analysts. Therefore some kind of institutionalized (but voluntary) mentor function for younger analysts would be most welcome. This might take the form of an offer for the new graduate to join a group or have contact with a senior and experienced analyst interested in supporting a younger colleague's personal development. Ideally, the mentor should stand independent of the institute's power functions.

Dewald has described how his admission to a training institute—let us presume that it was in connection with his being appointed as training analyst—gave a new perspective on his work insofar as earlier rigidities and fears of trying new techniques and theories diminished, leaving room for the integration of received knowledge in a more personal way (1997:74). Such is the result when "social rewards of diploma, prestige, and eventual inheritance of power are promised, rather than an opportunity to share an experience" (Dorn 1969:242). To my mind, it belongs to the more tragic aspects of psychoanalysis that being appointed as training analyst would be a precondition for the liberation of creativity.

6

CONCLUDING REFLECTIONS

In the previous chapter we investigated the disharmony between the ideals and values of psychoanalysis—the good that resides in its "intended ways"—and its way of organizing its institutions. This has been presented as a conflict between love and hate that has been built into the psychoanalytical project since its inception and up until our day. Thus, I find it reasonable to claim that the psychoanalytic institution still persists within the third epoch cited by Balint in his 1948 article. I have deemed it equally reasonable to describe some of this epoch's essential characteristics with the help of a heuristic model I call the superego complex.

What makes that protracted period (which has existed since the end of World War II) into a coherent epoch is that despite all the necessary insights, remarkably few changes have been implemented that would seriously alter that general structure that we perceive through the prism of the superego complex. I find the empirical foundation for such a statement in the fact that the analysis of the existing problems and the proposals for their remedy have, with very few exceptions, remained the same all the while. It is difficult to discern any essential difference between, for example, Balint's 1948 article, Bernfeld's paper from 1952 (published in 1962), and Kernberg's articles from 1986, 1996 or 2000.[1]

The overarching institutional problems, including authoritarian training structures, dictatorial training analysts, a general lack of theoretical curiosity, power struggles between rival

223

groups, and exaggerated expectations of supertherapies remain very much the same and are in the main still unsolved. The only really decisive reform within analytic training during this period has been the abandonment of the reporting system described in Chapter 4.

To capture this third epoch in a short formulation, I would say that it is *a time during which the psychoanalytic project has both submitted to and suffered under its institutions.*

It would seem reasonable to divide our following deliberations into two separate sections.

In the first, I will discuss what concerns the superego complex within psychoanalytic institutions. It is my conviction that, granted the political intention and courage, it would not take much time to remedy the institutional problems we have discussed in the last two chapters. There are, however, strong indications that such ambitions will soon grow and undergo radical changes during the next five or ten years. During the last decade, the IPA has taken various steps to analyze, initiate, and support necessary changes. Even if the political changes in some places may be quite dramatic, analytical institutions will surely have become different within the next five or fifteen years—on the condition, of course, that they will be allowed to survive at all.[2]

Another central factor in the production of necessary political ambition issues from the fact that psychoanalysis in our day exists in a time when societal changes are profound and take place at a pace making them more or less unsurveyable. These complications have been identified as "the crisis of psychoanalysis."

I will begin with the first perspective.

WHAT IS TO BE DONE?

Kernberg (1986) has published an analysis of the psychoanalytic training system's institutional problems in which he suggests four different models to help us envisage possible paths for the development of our existing training organizations.

The first of these models he names *the art academy*, the goal of which is to evoke the candidates' best qualities so that they may become good craftsmen or, at best, true artists of the psychoanalytic trade. This model is congruent with the analytic training system's individualized forms of teaching and also with prevalent notions of an ideal technique that must be skillfully managed for the analyst to attain the rank of Master. "Some psychoanalytic institutes, in fact, operate as if such an ideal technique, elevated to perfection by the local masters, existed and learning it from these masters is the best way for candidates to absorb and master it" (Kernberg 1986:807). However, psychoanalytic institutes do not function in the way that the ideal of an art academy presupposes: whereas, for example, a person teaching the art of painting openly will present his methods, the training analyst's technique is kept secret.

The second of Kernberg's models is *the technical* or *trade school*, where it is held that the primary goal of psychoanalytic training is to teach a clearly defined skill or profession, with no particular emphasis on artistry. Institutes of this kind, with a bureaucratic tendency, would establish an effective training program with close control over candidates' progress, ensuring graduation as soon as the expected skills have been acquired. Kernberg assumes that most analysts would object to such a model for the transmission of analytic proficiency. Nevertheless, this is the model most often met with when one surveys the training institutes in existence today—although modified in such a way that the criteria for acceptable skills are most often unclear and not very well accounted for. A more open organization would actually diminish the tendency for paranoid reactions.

Kernberg's third model for the psychoanalytic institute is *the monastery* or *religious retreat*. Here psychoanalysis is treated more or less like a system of religious beliefs. He maintains that whereas most analysts probably would reject such a model, there are, in fact, several clear elements in psychoanalytic training, as it is realized today, that actually correspond with it. Obvious instances of this tendency would be the idealization of theory and the mentors one has met with (e.g., the training analyst). Examples of this have been presented in the previous chapter.

Fourth, there is what Kernberg calls *the university college*, where education is offered by an institute with the task to promulgate and investigate knowledge together with the tools necessary for the creation of new knowledge. Within such a system, the candidate would not only be schooled in the history and development of theories and techniques, but also be exposed to prevalent critical discussion so that he may acquire the capacity to assess the different aspects of existing theory independently. In this way the candidate would be taught, within an atmosphere of scientific discussion, to contain and manage the multiplicity and uncertainty so prevalent today within the analytic community. When it comes to the election of institute staff within the university model, this would take place with openly declared criteria and procedures.

A model such as the university college, writes Kernberg, would most probably harmonize with the ideals of the average analyst, but all too seldom does it fit with the facts when one looks at the workings of actual psychoanalytic institutes. His conclusion is that there is a serious contradiction between goals and methods in the psychoanalytic training system: "While psychoanalytic educators think they are transmitting what is both an art and a science, they have structured their institutes so that they correspond most closely to a combination of the technical school and the theological seminary" (p. 812).

Kernberg suggests that the solution to this dilemma between ideals and realities must rest upon models of administration that actually tally with the pronounced goals of training. "In my view, the combined model of a university college and an art academy is the most promising for psychoanalytic education" (p. 827).

In what follows, I will make use of Kernberg's four models and, with their help, suggest some feasible steps aimed at correcting some of the ingrained institutional problems of psychoanalytic training. The suggestions—just like my whole investigation—are not primarily intended to better the pedagogy as such (that would have to be a project of its own), but are rather motivated by the hope of restricting the institutional foundations for a superego complex. Throughout, I will take for granted that such modifications are possible to realize under the prevailing circumstances that today surround the psychoanalytic project—*if there be* a sufficiently strong political intention.

To replace the tripartite Berlin model I suggest a *bipartite model of training* encompassing theoretical studies and clinical work under supervision. Personal analysis would remain only as a prerequisite for graduation.

We have seen that underlying existing institutional structures there has been an ambition that to a great extent is connected with the strivings of psychoanalysis to gain professional recognition. However necessary professionalization may have been to psychoanalysis and its goal to reach the status (albeit declining) it has today, its effects have not been merely good and the project as such may be heading toward conditions that will turn out to be quite impossible for the survival of the profession. With that in mind, the aim of the following suggestions is to suggest possible institutional structures that would primarily promote psychoanalysis as praxis in accordance with its "intended ways" (see Chapter 2).

It has been my intention to restrict the number of issues and keep to what seems to be most urgent. This is partly because present and historical realities within societies that are geographically dispersed differ to such an extent that it would be immodest and impractical to suggest any uniform and detailed program of change applicable to all. The diversification and experimentation of ideas is a positive trend that should be supported.

My suggestions link up with the analysis presented in Chapters 4 and 5. There is nothing really original in what I have to say; most of these ideas have been presented by others, some of them even long ago. What is unique will be apparent the day when decades of suggestions for radical change will finally be implemented.

Abolish the Training Analyst Institution

Interestingly enough, the existence of the training analyst as a separate but unofficial institution, during the very long period of its existence, has seldom been questioned (although with accelerating force during later years). (See "A State within the State" in Chapter 5). To liberate psychoanalytic institutional and organizational life from the burden of having such a condensed center of power, which in so many ways closes in on itself, would be one of the most important measures to take to lessen the ill effects of a superego complex: "What honesty is there in going along with [the institution of training analysts] if it is divisive, causes animosity, reinforces a feeling of failure, and is a factor producing society 'splits'?" (Aarons 1982–1983:686).

I therefore suggest a model in which candidates and possible candidates can have their personal analysis with any qualified analyst who has, say, five years of clinical experience and some five thousand sessions or so behind him. It would, in other words, be taken for granted that anyone who has gone through training and has matriculated is capable of conducting "good" psychoanalysis according to its "intended ways" (which would correspondingly imply that those who have been deemed unsuitable for the task have been removed from the training program or later expelled from their society).

That the newly graduated psychoanalyst is in need of years of further experience goes without saying—and hence the demand for a minimal number of years and sessions. Further than that, personal analysis cannot reasonably be other than "just as difficult or as easy as every other psychoanalysis. All that one needs to conduct the personal analysis of a colleague is the colleague's cooperation, some experience, and a lot of tact" Bernfeld 1962:482). Anything else would contribute to the further mystification of our profession (see below: "In Defense of a Wholly Independent Personal Analysis").

Allowing any experienced analyst in a society to conduct the personal analyses of candidates would considerably expand the group of conceivable training analysts, which, in smaller societies, would lessen any worries that resources to cover the need for training analyses will be lacking. Where the geographical conditions allow for it, I believe one could very well consider letting a prospective or actual candidate undertake his analysis with an analyst belonging to any other society maintaining the same training and quality requirements. The most important motive for such a change would not be to secure sufficient resources, but rather that a greater number of analysts with the authority to analyze (prospective) candidates would increase the possibility of keeping the personal analyses separate from seminars and supervisions. Maybe for the first time since the implementation of the Berlin model, a candidate would be allowed to experience his analysis as a truly personal one.[3]

The number of candidates an analyst should be allowed to have in analysis simultaneously should be restricted to, let us say, two so that possible tendencies for the formation of groups or convoys around certain individuals are diminished, together with the possibility of letting training analyses be a major source of income for a privileged group (something that is a reality in some societies today). And to be sure: no contact between the analyst and the institute—the analyst's sole obligation to report would be to sign a paper on which he specifies the duration and extent of the candidate's analysis to be presented when he wishes to graduate.

I have encountered the objection that if the training analyst institution were abolished the profession would be robbed of perhaps its one and only career path, something that is needed to attract gifted and ambitious individuals to the task. In response to this it could be argued that nowadays the position of training analyst is one of prestige only among analysts; the outside world most often understands nothing when one mentions that one is a training analyst. And in this lurks a danger, because the isolation of psychoanalysts in this respect may tempt them to inflate the status of training analyst to unrealistic proportions, which is just about what has actually happened.

The abolition of the training analyst institution may very well rob the profession of good possibilities of meriting its prominent members. In response to this I can only say that in such a case one will simply have to try harder and invent something different and better. The concentration of power and confidential information, together with the tendencies toward splitting that seem to follow inevitably from the training analyst institution, is wholly unacceptable for a business which, at least by implication, purports to have as one of its major goals to safeguard "the good" of psychoanalysis.

In line with the overarching aim of avoiding hierarchies between teachers and pupils beyond what is absolutely necessary, it is only reasonable that all formal differentiations in various groupings of different rank should be abolished altogether: "All relations between individuals must disintegrate into a contest of force unless there is universal agreement about the relative authority of all members; and the only terms on which such agreement seems possible among independent adult professionals is the assumption of their equality" (Guttman 1985:168). Thus we should abandon the system with "full members" and "associate members," which in different forms persists in many psychoanalytic societies (see note 7 to Chapter 5).

In Defense of a Wholly Independent Personal Analysis

Abandonment of the tripartite model in favor of one that is bipartite would mean that training proper would encompass only theoretical studies plus the supervised cases. (See "Didactic Analysis, Training Analysis, Personal Analysis" in Chapter 4.) In accordance with the suggestion to abolish the training analyst institution, what today goes under the rubric of training analysis would definitely transform into a personal analysis and nothing more. An analysis of that kind could then be either a requirement for admission to training or a necessary condition for graduation as a psychoanalyst, both of which surely must remain compulsory, without exception. The first option might be the best one, as it would make it more probable that the personal analysis is taken up out of a deeply felt need for help, which, at least to my mind, would be the only valid motive for anyone to want to grapple with the psychoanalytic experience.

Kovács makes the good observation that it is not time to let candidates meet their first patients until their main focus is directed toward the surrounding world and not at themselves (1936:351). Wouldn't the best personal analysis, then, be one that has been terminated before training begins? In the Paris Psychoanalytic Society, which actually has implemented the idea of a wholly personal analysis, it is required that an applicant shall have been in analysis preferably five and at least three years before being admitted to training (Szeczödy 1996, appendix 4, p. 4). If we are prepared to trust the capacity of candidates to arrive at independent evaluations and make wise decisions, we must also have confidence in their common sense, which would signal to them that if their supervised cases are running up against serious problems, they should seek analytical help once more.

The wish to enter psychoanalysis because of personal difficulties in living one's life must be counted as an important and positive prognostic criterion for someone who might one day become an analyst. If that requirement has been fulfilled and if the applicant has been in analysis with a sufficiently experienced analyst it must simply—in accordance with Guttman's way of reasoning (see above)—be assumed that the analytic experience has been "good enough." I therefore seriously question the demand that personal analysis take place during a part of or even during the entirety of the training process, which is a wholly unpsychoanalytical way of viewing things.

The transformation of the tripartite model of training into a bipartite one will bring a significant reduction of all exaggerated expectations with regard to the personal analysis; significantly, any notion of a supertherapy will be abjured.[4] I also believe that in line with all this, psychoanalytic institutions must in time accept that in the future, analyses taking place more than three times per week will most probably be the exception. With the seemingly inevitable social and economic developments taking place in our time it seems that all too few will have the means and/or the possibility to engage in psychoanalytic work four or five times a week. This would be just as applicable to "regular" analysands as to those who wish to undertake training. Therefore, to abandon the notion of a supertherapy entails the acceptance of the idea that a personal analysis must not necessarily be conducted with five sessions per week, although one might very well retain the requirement that the total number of sessions be some four or five hundred, as is the case in most societies today.[5]

As we have seen, the reporting system has, with one or two exceptions, disappeared. Nevertheless, it is not totally clear that an analyst should *under no circumstances whatsoever* be allowed to be present at or partake in the administrative or evaluative discussions that concern one of his analysands. In some institutes the procedure is that the candidate's analyst leave the room whenever his candidate is up for discussion. Such a rule should not only be upheld as a codex of honor, but be inscribed in the bylaws in such a way that *any* form of intervention be declared unethical: "Ideally it would seem best that the training analyst take no part in the administration and policy decisions of an institute. That is, those who undertake the personal analyses should not be supervisors or teachers" (Thompson 1958:49–50). Such an order of things will surely not, as if by magic, dispose of the difficulties connected with the analysis of (prospective) candidates, but would without doubt diminish such conflicts and difficulties.

Strengthen the Supervisory Function

As we have seen, it has almost always been taken for granted that anyone commissioned to be a training analyst is also suited to be a supervisor, which, to say the least, is a loose assumption. (See "The Supervised Cases" in Chapter 4.) As has been pointed out by so many, the abolition of the reporting system—and, reasonably, even more so the abolition of the training analyst institution together with the introduction of a bipartite training system—entails that the supervised cases be regarded as the central moment of training (and the supervisors as its most important functionaries). To meet this new reality some kind of formal qualification should be introduced for supervisors. The best way to do this would most probably be to implement a model that has been practiced in the Swedish Psychoanalytical Society since 1987, where anyone who wishes to supervise candidates first must pass a course for supervisors run by the institute (see note 41 to Chapter 4).

Anyone belonging to the same group of experienced analysts that has the right to conduct candidate analyses should be qualified to go through such a training. Some automatic screening should take place, as not all analysts are interested in supervision and will not apply, and some will discover during their attendance in the course that they lack interest or are simply not suited for the task. It is, however, extremely important that the supervisory function not become an opportunity to introduce yet another dividing hierarchy among psychoanalysts; therefore the institute should refrain from trying to direct which analysts should be allowed to belong to the group of supervisors. The risk that less well-suited individuals might become supervisors is, of course, a reality, but the danger of reinstating a new class system among analysts should motivate the institute to let things proceed according to their own ways. We can, I believe, trust that the "market forces" will let it be known which supervisors are the really good ones. The less suitable ones will soon be out of business.

So as not to subject the candidate to destructive infantilization, the choice of supervisor should be made wholly and genuinely voluntary so that the candidate is not only allowed to choose a supervisor from a list of those trained in his own institute or possibly at other institutes, but that he will also be free to select a new supervisor should the supervision not work satisfactorily. I believe this is an important point, because it seems that candidates switch supervisors much less often than one would expect, considering how very important it is that the supervisory pair be able to work creatively together. Some institutes follow the (most often unstated) rule that a candidate expressing dissatisfaction with his supervision is a problem and should be persuaded/forced to stay with the supervisor as long as it is at all feasible, while the hope is entertained that the problems at hand will be resolved in his personal analysis. That a candidate wishes to switch to another supervisor does not necessarily mean that the latter has failed. Supervision is a delicate task where the candidate finds himself in a vulnerable position; the fact that two persons under such conditions might find that they are not able to work optimally should surprise no one. It is much more important that the supervised case has the best possible support than that the institute act as if there could never be any reason for questioning members of its staff.

The therapeutic zeal that has come to expression as a syncretistic streak within the supervisory function must definitely be restrained—as when, for example, a supervisor admonishes his supervisee to clear up certain problems or issues in his personal analysis that have cropped up in supervision. I wish there were an explicit rule clearly repudiating any kind of act from members of the institute or supervisors that would be an attempt to influence the candidate's personal analysis, whether identified complications stem from the supervised cases or have to do with the candidate's general demeanor in his dealings with the institute or the society. Instead of telling the candidate to bring his difficulties somewhere else, the supervisor should be prepared to make them part of the supervision, without its being transformed into a new analysis. He should also stay open to the effect his own personality and style may have upon the candidate's possibilities for learning during their interaction (Berman 2000).

In my experience, the detailed clinical theories so often taught in psychoanalytic institutes can easily disturb the candidate's intuitive and emotional perception. Supervisors may at times find it difficult to communicate concerning their analysands in a way that is not dominated by the candidate's need or request for applying the newly acquired knowledge, which, in most cases, will alienate him from his analysand due to the purely technical approach that will easily take over.

When institutes completely give up the ambition to control via the training analysis, the candidate is offered a wholly new mandate to decide *for himself* whether, in the light of his self-awareness, he believes he will one day become a good-enough analyst. We should profit from this concept and let candidates be involved in their own evaluation!

Cremerius refers to the "open" institutional forms practiced within the Canadian, French, and Swiss societies as a model:

> Here, it is the candidate's task to acquire psychoanalytical experience and proficiency through a personal analysis, through supervision, and through participation in lectures and seminars. It is his responsibility to demonstrate that he has become an analyst. This he will do by presenting a clinical case to a committee and defend his theses. The institute will take no responsibility for his education. [Cremerius 1987:1092; see also Thomä 1993:17–19; A.-M. Sandler 1982:391].[6,7]

Make Room for Theoretical Work and Necessary Research

Kernberg (2000:112) suggests that we redefine the task of psychoanalytical institutes and turn them into producers of new ana-

lytical knowing, a concept I interpret as an extension of his earlier suggestion that we might best view psychoanalytic training
as a mixture of the university and the art academy (1986:827).[8]
(See "The Theoretical Seminars" in Chapter 4.)

The university aspect of the combination model should not
be taken as a proposal for joining analytical training to the university. A number of discussants on this issue have suggested such
a solution, but I would rather see that the university model be a
guideline for the theoretical seminars and for the management and
transmission of psychoanalytical knowing. In this way psychoanalytic institutes can liberate themselves from the notion that
their task is to teach a doctrine, with the entailing danger that
training becomes a form of indoctrination. Theoretical studies
should rather have as their aim to provide an experience that will
lay the foundation for the prospective analyst's capacity for conducting theoretical work (see Chapter 2) by reflecting upon received knowledge, evaluating it for himself, and to some extent
also producing new knowledge.

Arlow has pointed out how psychoanalysis has taken upon
itself the mission to train new analysts without any clear or organized theory for the learning process (1982:6). Therefore we must
start experimenting with pedagogical forms that are suited to meet
the needs of adult students, and not devised for the education of
children.[9] One way of doing this would be to break up the conventional system of the Berlin model with its fixed curriculum
designed to secure a specified and controlled acquisition of knowledge. Instead we should—as does happen in some institutes
today (see Kernberg 2000)—try alternative models with a variety
of courses and seminars for candidates to choose from, with only
a minimal compulsory curriculum, the latter, on the one hand, so
that a group of candidates accepted for training will not risk splitting up in totally separate monads, and on the other, because certain basic knowledge is indispensable for conducting a dialogue
among the members of the profession. Perhaps the compulsory
part should take up about 30 or 40 percent of the time allotted for
theoretical studies.[10]

Depending on the prevailing conditions in the area, I imagine that institutes would try to establish as large an offering as possible of high-quality seminars dealing with topics and issues relevant for both clinical and theoretical work. Encourage analysts, in consultation with the institute, to start seminars dealing with topics that engage them. There is probably no better form for transmission of analytical knowing than having experienced analysts share their clinical work with a group of candidates in the spirit of the art academy.[11] Conjoin the output of seminars with that of other analytic (or psychotherapeutic) institutes in the region. Here are not only synergistic rewards to be gained, but also new and sometimes unexpected paths for widening the scope of theoretical work. Of course, some seminars can, and perhaps even should, be held in collaboration with the university; certain topics —such as the history of psychoanalysis, its metascience and research issues, its relations with other disciplines (such as philosophy, neuropsychology, cognitive psychology, etc.), ethical and legal issues—can very well be handled within a purely academic milieu.[12]

Where strict considerations of confidentiality are not an obstacle, the freely chosen seminars should be open not only to candidates but also to graduated analysts within the society. In a wider perspective we might experiment with inviting persons rooted in other disciplines and activities who may be expected to contribute essential knowledge and experience. In this way, and to a much greater extent, the training of candidates will become a concern for the society as a whole, which in turn would diminish the tendency of the institute to defend and preserve a hegemonic position for its elite and its doctrine.

The best way of promoting an open and presuppositionless atmosphere between analytic colleagues would certainly be to sustain such a spirit during the training process. Therefore it is important not to reject challenging and intellectually experienced applicants—on the condition, of course, that there is a true preparedness to receive and embrace such assets and not just kill them with silence, as seems to happen so often.

The ambition to create a more academic relationship to knowledge in connection with theoretical studies would be one step toward abandoning the notion that psychoanalytic knowledge is a cumulative mass (in accordance with an obsolete but in many quarters still tacitly cherished conception of a unitary science). It is, however, a steadily growing and widespread conviction that psychoanalysis should perhaps not firsthandedly be thought of as a science, at least in a purely empirical-positivistic sense. Even when one is not prepared to say exactly what psychoanalysis may *be* precisely, it must—when such an insight is taken seriously—take a new stance in relation to its own knowing.

At the end of Chapter 4 I pointed out how ambivalent psychoanalysis is in its way of relating to its own knowledge. On the one hand an obvious dependency upon knowledge is noticeable, and on the other it treats knowledge—and not least theoretical work—with some condescension. Making room for theoretical work is not primarily a question of creating new structures within the organizations and institutions, but rather of leaving space for freer thinking. This may sound like a vague suggestion, and in fact it is, until that juncture where ideals are to be transformed into reality. There are no preestablished models to lean against, and whatever solution one chooses, it must be implemented in accordance with prevailing local and historical conditions.

What then concerns research proper as distinguished from theoretical work? There are so many urgent issues to be dealt with that it would be impossible to try to deal with them extensively here. One area that has been much under discussion during the last ten to fifteen years, due to the present political and economic conditions in Europe and the United States, is investigation into the efficacy of the treatment that psychoanalysts offer, that is to say quantitative or qualitative research on the meaningfulness—in terms of actual (albeit perhaps too often psychiatrically defined) results—of psychoanalysis and psychoanalytically oriented psychotherapy. To communicate with third-party financiers and politically controlled institutions psychoanalysis will have to depend upon statistical and empirical research, which in our day seems to be the only way to determine which propositions may be judged trustworthy.

Other—and for psychoanalysis itself perhaps more pertinent—areas of research would touch upon such issues as events within the analytic/psychotherapeutic process, the role of psychoanalysis in a time of great changes, the effects of differing models of training, and so on. As to the last point, the IPA has already promoted the evaluation of experimenting so that new findings may be available to all societies.[13]

Finally, some kind of reward system for meritorious theoretical work and scientific production that will stand free from all functions of power must be created. That would stimulate both analysts and candidates to take an interest in psychoanalytic knowing in general and in theoretical work in particular.

Make Training More Accessible

Something of a revolution took place in the United States in conjunction with the judicial ruling in 1989 that nonmedical clinical practitioners (among them psychologists) be allowed to enter training within APA institutes and subsequently seek membership. From a European point of view this may have seemed to be a marginal event. There, at least psychologists have almost always had access to analytic training.

The aptitude for becoming a good analyst only rarely coincides with the aptitude for being accepted to medical or psychological education. It would therefore seem reasonable to try to attract possible applicants for analytic training from other areas. In that respect there are strong traditions to draw from. England (something similar exists in France) has always welcomed those who seem suitable and who can be expected to live up to the demands of the training system (even though the quota is kept low enough to ensure that physicians remain in the majority—more of that below). Thus we find analysts there who are philosophers, doctors of literature, social workers, clergymen, and so forth.

Allowing new groups to enter the profession is one of many ways of diversifying not only training itself but also the analytical community as a whole—of which it is in dire need. It may be contended that according to tradition or even law it may be impossible to conduct psychoanalysis by so-called laymen when it is considered to be an integral part of the medical establishment's set of measures, thereby controlling it with legislation on certification and quackery. That issue is as yet insufficiently investigated, and if psychoanalysis should ever loosen its bonds with medicine it may very well happen that it defines itself in a way making it possible for it to operate outside of the bounds of medical legitimacy.

Finally: bring in younger candidates. The tendency has unfortunately been to choose candidates based upon their earlier experience and competence within the psychotherapeutic field. Choosing candidates among the most experienced psychotherapists will, of course, result in the average age being rather high. Negative effects issuing from this have been discussed earlier.

Make Power More Transparent

Power and its exercise are unavoidable in any society or training system that must be managed with efficiency, but within psychoanalytic institutes power has tended to become overly diffuse and inaccessible through hidden management procedures and features like the training analyst institution. (See "A State within the State" in Chapter 5.) Based on the suggestion above that we should strive to establish a state of affairs concerning the relative authority of analysts founded on the presupposition that all are equal, we should seek to attain the greatest possible openness in bylaws and practice.

Let the overarching policy for psychoanalytic training be an issue for the members of the society to agree upon by ballot. Full openness should be the rule when it comes to requirements, criteria, and routines pertaining to the institute's handling of all candidate issues (but certainly with total confidentiality in individual cases). Let all forms and standards for evaluation and decision making in connection with selection, graduation, complaints, or expulsion of a candidate be openly accounted for and open for continual discussion. Appoint all positions within both society and institute in the same way that available offices are announced in government institutions. Clear and overt criteria will define the group of possible applicants.

Following such a model it should not be difficult to establish systems with reasonably just appointments to office and a meaningful level of member control of the institute's activities.

PSYCHOANALYSIS AND ITS UNCERTAIN FUTURE

The claim that we still live in the third epoch of the psychoanalytic institution is in no way intended to deny that in other important respects—that is to say, outside the sphere demarcated and marked by the general structure of the superego complex—this has been a very dynamic period. The third epoch cannot be said to have been homogeneous and without development. Despite the stubborn survival of the superego complex, there has been a considerable lessening of orthodoxy and self-proclaimed authority. During the seventies, American psychoanalysis could not ignore the fact that there was no longer the same request for it coming from psychiatry, while at the same time this was the beginning of a period of extensive diversification, both clinically and theoretically, which is still going on.[14] On the whole, a vital sense of openness seems to have spread within the psychoanalytic movement.[15] One of the great changes for American psychoanalysis has also been the fact that the center of gravity for psychoanalysis has gradually shifted from the United States to England.[16]

In the fifties and sixties one would every now and then come across articles in the analytic publications with titles like "Psychoanalysis Today" or "The Present Status of Psychoanalysis." For certain, the kind of worry was aired that easily breeds within a discipline that is closed to the surrounding world and in many quarters so poorly regarded as is psychoanalysis. Yet, the general impression from these texts is that we are continually and anew summing up and celebrating its successes after World War II. However, with the growing realization that we are no longer the pet discipline of psychiatry, the tone has changed, and in later years we have devoted considerable time and energy to discussing the current problems of psychoanalysis.

During the years 1988–1990 nine articles were published in the *Psychoanalytic Quarterly* under some kind of variation of the rubric "The Future of Psychoanalysis,"[17] and the two fundamental issues reappearing in these contributions were "What will our profession look like in the future?" and "What will psychoanalytic theories of the mind and its treatment be like?" Even though it is possible to discern a certain sense of crisis in these articles, they are mostly characterized by their wonder regarding the future. However, just a few years later, the sense of crisis was much more apparent.

In 1994 the newly formed House of Delegates within the IPA had established a committee with the mission to investigate the widespread view among the component societies that psychoanalysis was in a state of crisis. In the report presented a year later (RHDC 1995), it was abundantly clear that within a majority of the world's societies there was an acute sense of crisis.

By now, there is a whole row of elements perceived to be part of this crisis. A summary of these could look something like this:

> *A drastic reduction during the past twenty years or so of the number of applicants for analytic treatment*, one of the results of which is that nowadays psychoanalysts are engaged in psychoanalytic work at a much lower level than before. This state of affairs is partly attributable to worsened economic conditions, but it has been reported that even when analysis is offered with strongly reduced fees or almost gratis— as is the case with analysis with candidates in some institutes—it is still difficult to recruit analysands.

Parallel to this, *psychoanalysis of today suffers much tougher com-*
petition from other methods for treating mental problems.
Despite its long-standing dialogue with psychoanalysis,
psychiatry has in later years resolutely come to define itself in purely medical and biological terms. Today it feels
triumphant as it celebrates the last ten to twenty years of
advancement within the area of psychopharmacology.
Within the psychotherapeutic sphere, new forms of behavior therapy, together with cognitive psychotherapy, are
increasingly replacing psychoanalysis and psychodynamic
therapies as psychiatry's prime allies.

To the extent that it is still possible to practice psychoanalysis,
third-party funding has increased considerably. Most often
this will mean that some private medical insurance or social security system will be paying the bills, rather than the
analysand taking the money from his own pocket. To what
extent total or partial coverage will take place does, of
course, vary. One serious result of this has been that analytic confidentiality risks being compromised when the
paying party (understandably) wishes to have some degree
of control over the planning and surveillance of the treatment process.

Today, however, the increasing trend seems to be that
third-party funding is withdrawing from offering any support
for psychoanalytic treatment. Differing systems of buying psychoanalytic and psychotherapeutic services on the market have
the common effect of forcing analysts to compete with each
other, leading to lower fees and economic deterioration.

There are fewer applicants to the analytic training institutes.
Psychiatry's weakened confidence in psychoanalysis makes
physicians less prone to seek analytic training (and the risk
that psychoanalysis should no longer be dominated by the
medical profession has been perceived by many as a serious threat). One important factor behind the diminishing
influx is, of course, impaired economic conditions, another
one is brought up in the next item.

There currently exists weakened legitimacy for psychoanalysis. The last ten to twenty years has seen a steady flow of more or less well-founded critique and at times more bloodthirsty attacks aimed at psychoanalysis, a phenomenon that has been called "Freud-bashing" and that at least in part seems to be a response to the claim of psychoanalysis that it is a science, something that unfortunately has made it an easy target of criticism. Besides the purely epistemological and philosophical bases for such critique, there has also been the pressure coming from an increasingly strong and pervasive biologism, an ideological current founded upon the great advances made by disciplines such as genetics and neurology during the last decades of the twentieth century.

In addition to this comes a strongly experienced inability of psychoanalysis to define its knowing and its practice in a way that makes it meaningful to new times, and a form of social, political, and historical development about which almost everyone—not just analysts, but also sociologists, historians, economists, and even futurologists—still seems to be groping in the dark when it comes to understanding its essence.

Beyond such external factors, there are also *the persisting existence and effects of the superego complex*, which has been investigated in this book: a training system that in many respects is antiquated, together with the destructive forms of cohabitation within the institutions. As Bollas says in an interview: "Psychoanalysis just has to survive 'the psychoanalytic movement.' If it survives psychoanalysts and their schools, then it will grow and develop. But this remains to be seen" (quoted in Molino 1997:50).

But that is not all, for even the future of psychoanalytic institutions themselves is uncertain. To say just a little concerning this, I would like to bring up two possible scenarios that have to do with changes in the economic conditions for psychoanalysts and psychoanalysis itself.

We have seen how the possibilities for analysts to practice have gradually diminished. As psychoanalysts will have to find other ways of generating an income, for example from short or long psychotherapies, or even find it outside their offices, this will affect not only individual analysts, but psychoanalysis itself.

It is relatively easy to become an analyst, whereas it is becoming increasingly difficult to patch things together so that one may sustain oneself as a practicing one, where learned skills may not only be maintained but also allowed to deepen and mature. An analyst is defined by the fact that he sees analysands, and in the previous chapter we saw how very important are the first ten years of an analyst's professional life. For him to be able to develop his competence and skills it is required that he be immersed in analytical work for a number of years. How will the newly graduated analyst even come close to the number of sessions required for this to happen if he cannot find analysands?

When circumstances do force him to abandon his praxis, he will gradually change into something other than a psychoanalyst. How, then, will psychoanalysis survive when there is no longer a group large enough to transmit psychoanalytic knowing by the institutional forms of analyzing candidates and supervising them? It should be apparent that these troublesome issues and problems completely stand apart from any issue concerning the existence or nonexistence of the training analyst or the superego complex. Things are simply much too urgent for that.

Narrowing financial conditions, as dictated by lessening demand from the general public and a much more frugal treatment by third-party financial providers, will sooner or later influence psychoanalytic institutions. The unemployment among the ranks of psychoanalysts today is only scantily concealed through their ability to dedicate themselves to other tasks, such as psychotherapy, supervision and organizational development, research, psychiatry and so on.

But, in line with this, analysts' incomes will to a lesser degree come from their private firms. This will reduce the will and capacity to pay the high fees connected with affiliation to professional institutions when these costs have to be covered with money from an income that has already been taxed.

It has been discussed whether analysts should reduce their fees to recover at least some part of the number of analytic hours they once were accustomed to having. Should this strategy be successful in terms of more analysands, the problem with the funding of analytical institutions still remains when the financial base is diminished. In the long run it may then be presumed that analytic institutions will shrink, not just because of economic limitations, but also because the number of potential candidates is diminishing. With that, the institutionally founded psychoanalytical authority would also dwindle, perhaps even to the point where it is no longer possible to maintain institutes and training systems of the kind described in this book.

I should also, in this connection, mention the phenomenon of the obvious theoretical diversification within the psychoanalytic movement during the last thirty to forty years. As we have seen, the reactions to this development have been diverse. Even if we do welcome theoretical diversity—something I defend in Chapter 2—we must be aware that underneath sudden flare-ups of interest in new theoretical foundations there must be some kind of suspicion toward established views, which is part of the crisis of psychoanalysis. In diversification there is always an inherent centrifugal force which, in the empty space that would arise should analytic institutions be on the decline, would engender tendencies toward splitting.

So, with weakened psychoanalytic institutions, less centralized control, and a possible inherent centrifugal force, one might expect a tendency toward dispersion within the analytical movement, where new groups with locally developed organizational forms would evolve.

I believe that this should not be perceived as only a negative scenario. I also believe that it would be very detrimental to psychoanalysis if it were to lose institutions like the IPA and the IFPS. Their authority has, for better or worse, offered the best guarantee for the relative unity of the psychoanalytic project.[18] But a psychoanalytic movement with a preserved institutional center—albeit having a different structure than what we have been used to—striving to maintain a vital dialogue with an analytic periphery, would, in my judgment, have a lot to gain. There are signs today that this is the very direction in which we are heading.

Psychoanalysis has been moving toward a point where the position it enjoyed within American and European culture for more than half a century—a period when the superego complex of the third epoch was characteristic of its inner life—no longer is available to it. Some take the changes of our times to be signs that we cannot even be sure if there will be any psychoanalysis at all in thirty or fifty years.[19] To others, present developments carry a promise of positive changes on the condition that we succeed in dealing with the underlying problems.

So, even to someone who chooses a more optimistic stance it would seem most probable that what we today refer to as "the crisis of psychoanalysis" will stand out in the future as a period of decisive change in its development. Whatever this may entail, it should be clear that the conditions for protection and support from the surrounding society will be radically different, that analysands will show up with new expectations from psychoanalysis, and that analysis itself will in all probability have to reflect on its own activities and institutions along radically new lines. We may well wonder whether this will not become one of the most important tasks for the future: to produce a discourse capable of demonstrating how psychoanalysis—which, after all, has been formed by its having developed within a modernistic context—is able to respond to urgent needs arising also within a context of late (or post-) modernism.

End Notes

Chapter 1

1. My notion of an analytic superego was in no way original. The superego is a central psychoanalytic concept that was widely used in analytical reflection soon after its introduction. Thus, Michael Balint wrote that what we need is "a new orientation of our training system which must aim less at establishing a new and firm super-ego but more at enabling the candidate to free himself and to build up a strong ego which shall be both critical and liberal at the same time" (Balint 1948:171). Several later authors have written of the analyst's superego, both as a wished-for and an unwanted effect of training.

2. Since the middle of the eighties, the set of rules regulating training are quite similar in both the internationals.

Chapter 2

1. My notion of a good that cannot be addressed with abstract formulations, but only discovered through the medium of practice is, as far as I am able to judge, congruent with Arendt's exposition of the Aristotelian conception of virtue (*arete*): Virtues are not taken to be abstract capacities "manifesting themselves." Instead, virtue should be understood to be *active action* (praxis), which is to say that *the good or virtue is inherent in the very execution of an act* and is not its precondition (Arendt 1958:207).

A more modern metaphysic would suggest that virtue is tantamount to the *capacity* to realize a certain goal, as if it were a personal *quality*. It is from such conceptions that one will try to assemble a catalogue to cover the virtues.

2. I differentiate between an interactional and an intersubjective perspective. The former—like the notion of an "interpersonal" space, or, for that matter, the object relations theory—is based on a conception of two separate subjects who are objects (representations) to each other; the latter rests on the

assumption of a fundamental intersubjectivity preceding any differentiation between subject and object. What thus may not have been recognized by the adherents of the intersubjective model is that an object relations theory will not fully match the comprehension of the analytic relationship proposed by the model. Even though object relations theory—in its varied forms—has been of enormous import for the development of psychoanalytic knowledge and technique, it does suffer from some significant limitations, even in regard to its goal of offering a fresh view of the analytical relationship as such. This is not the place to critique the object relations theory, so I restrict myself to pointing out how it fails to account for a truly intersubjective axis of communication. For, as we saw, object relations theory will only be able to depict a relationship between subjects and their objects, the latter being wholly constituted in the realm of representation. In other words, it can only account for the intrasubjective *idea* of the Other, but not *the Other as such*, in his or her enigmatic and evanescent presence. Thus, object relations theory knows only a mediated intersubjectivity, but not intersubjectivity of the first degree. To approximate something of the kind, it must resort to concepts such as "projective identification" (see Ogden 1979), which, when used to cover the area of intersubjectivity, tends to become a bit stretched.

Dunn (1995) summarizes several of the central trains of thought, presents the main authors, and provides a first critique of the intersubjective view (see also Jacobs 1999).

3. See Reeder 1996 and 1998b for an exposition of the theoretical basis for my use of the term "interpreting."

4. In *Reflecting Psychoanalysis* (Reeder 1996:191–192) I suggested the notion of a "matrix of transference," a term I had borrowed from Winnicott (1958:33). The matrix of communication—a concept inspired by Heidegger's category *Mitsein*, Being-with (see Heidegger 1927:§26)—is my theoretical extension of the matrix of transference, with a wider area of application that may be of value for the introduction of the latter. I would like to elevate the "with" intended in *Mitsein* above connotations such as "together with" to a "pure" or even "metaphysical" "with" as *a "common presence" that precedes all "coming together" between subjects consciously aware of one another.*

5. For a detailed survey of the phenomenon of countertransference from Freud until our day, see Jacobs 1999.

6. The Swedish expression here is *skitunge*, which literally means "shitty" or "dirty" child. It is an expression meant only in jest and has in fact a rather endearing quality.

7. My exposition of analytic interpreting has been inspired by Schön's theory of reflection-in-action (Schön 1983; see also Schön 1987).

8. The kind of capacity I am trying to capture with expressions like "faith in the Other" or "awaiting" are, in the analytic literature, most probably clos-

est to W. R. Bion's idea that the analyst's task is "to be one with O" (Bion 1970). If one might find Bion's formulation a bit laconic, mine may be of some help.

9. The distinction between *knowing* and *knowledge* is borrowed from the one often made in French between *savoir* and *connaissance*. Knowing pertains to the (unconscious, primary process) *disposition* or *capacity* for saying or doing, whereas knowledge has to do with *contents* residing in the (conscious, secondary process) mind, such as may be expressed in the form of propositional statements. Thus, knowledge will always presuppose knowing, but not necessarily the other way around.

10. The issues discussed here have been brought up in a similar manner in an article by Parsons (1992), in which he strives to cast some light on the interactional relationship psychoanalysts have with their theories. Parsons takes as a point of departure a text by Joseph Sandler (1983), where it is maintained that the analyst possesses unexpressed (preconscious) segments of theory that are not necessarily congruent or compatible with generally accepted (clinical) theory, but that offer a background for his understanding and interpreting.

Whereas Parsons perhaps is more "phenomenologically" descriptive in his approach, my attempt is to dissect the processes through which theoretical knowledge transforms into clinical competence. Also, whereas Parsons stresses the refinding of unexpressed theoretical standpoints, I rather suggest that what takes place here is more like the invention of something new.

11. Andrew Brook (1992) has proposed the idea that psychoanalytic theory is a continuation of commonsense psychology.

12. It is only when we fully formalize our theories—after the model of mathematics or logic—that we are spared this demand. On the other hand, comprehensibility will decrease rapidly if we should choose such a solution, and any interpretation of the formulae thus engendered will necessitate narrative exposition anyhow.

13. Together with the capacity to *endure ignorance* for shorter or longer periods of time, this is, to me, the most radical interpretation of Bion's suggestion that the analyst in every encounter with the analysand receive him without memory, desire, understanding, or knowledge (Bion 1967, 1970). My idea is the same as Bion's, with the possible addition that I lay greater stress on *invention* as such.

Chapter 3

1. Winter (1999) offers a thorough description of the ideological foundations for the professionalization process of psychoanalysis, together with the institutionalization of its system of knowledge. (There is also an interesting description of Freud's strategies for the development of an authoritative rendering of the meaning of psychoanalysis.) For a depiction of psychoanalysis

as a profession before it established a fixed curriculum of professionalization, see Falzeder 2000.

2. To begin with, the clinic announced its existence through advertisements in the papers, which sufficed to attract a considerable number of applicants. Soon enough the message started to spread through those who had visited the clinic (Oberndorf 1926:320).

3. Attempts had actually been made to shorten analytic sessions at the clinic from 60 minutes, which at that time was the norm, to 30. However, this proved feasible only with a select choice of patients and therefore one offered 45 or the hour's full 60 minutes three to four times a week. (See Eitingon 1923:262).

4. The early psychoanalytic movement was inspired by a social—not to say socialistic—pathos in a way that would be quite uncharacteristic after World War II. For details concerning this tendency within the movement and its deplorable suppression, see Jacoby 1983.

5. See also Eitingon 1925 on the importance of the control analysis.

6. In a report from the ITC by Edward Bibring in 1938, these events are mentioned quite summarily with the wording that the Berlin Institute "has been incorporated with other therapeutic bodies in a central organization" (1938:272).

7. For an analysis of the ideological and practical inheritance from the Berlin Institute to analytic training, see Cremerius 1986.

8. For a detailed presentation of the evolution of the Vienna Clinic, its tasks, plus political and social aspirations, see Danto 1998.

9. My description of the events is incomplete. One would have to wade through oceans of minutes, reports, and articles, together with published and unpublished correspondence, to correctly capture the delicate processes taking place at this time, events that have been decisive for later developments within the psychoanalytic movement. Thus, I limit myself to a simplified narrative on the basis of various documents that I have happened to stumble upon.

10. For a condensed rendering of the organizational evolution of American psychoanalysis from the second decade of the twentieth century until World War II, see Pollock 1961:484–485.

11. The whole sequence of events alluded to here is described in detail by Jones (1957).

12. For a more detailed description of the two standpoints closer to our own day, see Fischer 1982.

13. This conflict was handsomely hidden within the reports coming from the ITC—as if one didn't want to believe that there was a real contradiction at hand. In his ITC report of 1939, Edward Glover wrote diplomatically that "it was resolved to leave *the adjustment of relations* between the American Psycho-Analytic Association and the I.T.C. in the hands of the Committee or of the

Business Meeting of the International Psycho-Analytical Association" (1939:212; my italics).

14. Whereas Balint's article is a given item in any list of literature dealing with psychoanalytic training and its development, Szasz's brilliant analysis is most often omitted. I presume this would have to do with how Szasz—with his indisputable intellectual honesty—convincingly exposes the internal claims for power within the analytical movement and the authoritarian order it subjugates its members to. In a paper from 1966, Leo Rangell, at the time president of the IPA, states laconically and within parentheses that "Szasz is not *all* wrong" (1967:427, italics in original).

15. For a penetrating study of one such (and ill-fated) case, see Paul Roazen's (1969) *Brother Animal: The Story of Freud and Tausk*.

16. For a historical survey of orthodoxy within the psychoanalytic movement, see Bergmann 1997.

17. Ian Parker (1997:186) maintains that the Lacanian movement is the most widely disseminated and well-organized psychoanalytic "school" in the world today. For a closer look at the Lacanian movement's peculiar mixture of constant splitting and rigid organization, see Roudinesco 1993.

The extended process whereby Lacan was finally excluded from the IPA is depicted in Miller (1977). For an interesting contemporary image of the relations between IPA and the international Lacanian movement that has evolved since Lacan's death in 1981, see the discussions held in 1996 in Buenos Aires between the then-president of the IPA, Horacio Etchegoyen, and the Lacanian movement's foremost but certainly not undisputed representative, Jacques-Alain Miller (Etchegoyen and Miller 1996).

18. Ego psychology was developed in the United States during the thirties, forties, and fifties by the German immigrants Heinz Hartmann, Ernst Kris, Rudolf Loewenstein, Edith Jacobson, and others.

19. This short history is based mainly on Knight 1953, Szasz 1958, and Bird 1968.

20. As just one example of a place where the position of psychoanalysis would have been different if this connection did not exist I could mention the financing of treatment with an analyst who is a physician, which for almost three decades was provided by the Swedish social security system, but which is now on the decline. In the wake of this system analysands with psychologist analysts could, for about half that time, rely upon different (although weaker) forms of support. Today social financing of analysis with psychologists in Sweden is practically nonexistent.

21. For an illuminating survey of the position of psychoanalysis in American social life in the middle of the 1960s, see Berger 1965.

22. For a description of the authority of American medicine at this time and its relation to psychoanalysis, see Eisold 1998:874–876.

23. For an illustrative depiction of the extent to which American psycho-analysis was intertwined with psychiatry, see "Minimal Standards for the Training of Physicians in Psychoanalysis," in the *Bulletin of the American Psychoanalytic Association* 1956: 12/714–721. See also Levin and Michaels 1961.

24. Cf.: "To the extent that the image, *psychoanalyst*, became a repository for unanalyzed infantile hopes and aspirations, psychoanalytic training inadvertently may have appeared to offer a 'royal road' to fantasy fulfillment rather than to acknowledgment, awareness and working through of unresolved infantile problems. To the candidate and new member who expected to find a utopian existence, psychoanalysis failed to accomplish its main potential benefit" (Dorn 1969:246–247, italics in original).

25. See also Gitelson 1956 and Menninger 1956. For a personal depiction of an American psychiatrist's road to psychoanalysis during and just after World War II, see Dewald 1997:69–73.

26. See Gitelson 1956.

27. To a great extent marked by its aspiration to remain a purely descriptive empirical discipline, psychiatry has been lacking a language of its own for interpreting the human condition (there have been exceptions, such as Karl Jaspers, Ludvig Binswanger, or Medard Boss, beautiful anomalies who never managed to leave more than evanescent traces). This has made it predisposed to devoting large portions of its intellectual energy to different taxonomic systems in an attempt to at least classify the world even when it is not possible to speak of it.

In addition, it has struggled with great difficulties to develop effective treatments; not until chlorpromazine was on the market in the fifties did any really meaningful alternative appear to the often cruel methods that had reigned earlier and that seem to be taken straight from the horror shop of the asylum: restraints, straitjackets, hydrotherapies, electrotherapies, sterilizations, lobotomies, and so on. For want of a proper language and effective treatment modalities, and with greater or lesser enthusiasm, at least parts of the psychiatric establishment have assimilated psychoanalytic concepts and methods during a large portion of the twentieth century, but practically never without redefining the concepts or integrating them within contexts that have made them lose much of their original meaning.

One important factor underlying this development was the welfare ideology for modern society that evolved at about the same time. The American welfare ideology has in many respects differed from the European one, and alongside a rapid expansion of social engineering and social work, it came to expression as a movement for psychiatric reform sooner than in Europe. Influential parts of the psychiatry that developed under the aegis of a welfare ideology—that is to say, those parts that were not markedly biologically oriented, but instead rested upon an American psychiatric tradition with its roots in the "moral therapy" of the nineteenth century—were at the time in need of a more modern theory and human ideal. It therefore took to heart the implicit humanistic values of psychoanalysis together with its ambition to understand human suffering and not respond just with purely medical interventions. Thus evolved dynamic psychiatry, which for all intents and purposes remained a medically oriented psychiatry, albeit animated with psychoanalytic knowledge and clinical methodology.

28. Ekstein and Wallerstein's classical study, *The Teaching and Learning of Psychotherapy* (1958), gives a picture of the psychiatric milieus where psychotherapy and psychoanalysis tended to be intermixed. In our day it is the rule rather than the exception that anyone applying for psychoanalytic training already has an established identity as a psychotherapist. How this tends to influence psychoanalytic training and the psychoanalyst's professional development is discussed in Joseph and Wallerstein 1982.

29. For a description of the evolution of American dynamic psychiatry, see Gitelson 1951 and 1962b.

30. For a long period the William Alanson White Institute in New York was a center of power within the IFPS. In later years a power shift has taken place in favor of the European component societies; in particular the Swedish and Finnish societies have been prominent.

For a personal view on the IFPS' specific qualities and importance in the psychoanalytic world, see Rodrigues 1999.

31. For a variegated description of the American psychologists' struggle to gain access to training programs certified by the IPA, see Lane and Meisels 1994. For a shorter version, see Wallerstein 1998a and for a more extensive version, see Wallerstein 1998b.

Chapter 4

1. One can only agree with what Nielsen wrote in the fifties: "Analysis ought to be begun early in life, a demand which unfortunately seems to run contrary to present trends" (1954:249).

2. See, for example Cremerius 1986, Fliess 1942, Greenacre 1961, Heimann 1968, Kappelle 1996, Sharpe 1947, Thomä 1993, Van Der Leeuw 1962.

3. Only a few years previously, Van Der Leeuw's compatriot, Lampl-De Groot, had written the following: "[W]e prefer to reject an applicant rather than to educate inefficient persons. A small group of efficient workers is more valuable than a large group of mediocre members" (1954:185).

4. Some American discussants have suggested defining the analyst's desired qualities in terms of ego functions—as if an ego psychological perspective would give a more scientifically objective picture of what an analyst ought to be! Greenacre reports that at the beginning of the sixties analysts in Chi-

cago supported research on such ego functions, she herself stating the reservation that there is something to this model that makes of the whole selection process a simple employment procedure (1961:51–52). The project never resulted in a new and epoch-making process of selection, but it did engender some interesting material. For a thorough analysis of the various facets of selection and suggestions for further research in the field, see, for example, Pollock 1976. See also C.E.A. 1978, where the same restriction is formulated as seems to be agreed upon today: "At present we question whether it is possible with any certainty to say more than the following: that a person who seems analysable, says he wants to be an analyst, and has accomplished in life enough so far to give promise that he can carry out what he intends to do or wants to be, should be acceptable" (p. 84). See also Holt and Luborsky 1955.

5. Thomä (1993:17–18) mentions a "genius paragraph" in Austrian legislation of psychotherapy which, to ensure access to the uniquely endowed, makes *anyone* with special gifts who would be suited for the task eligible for psychoanalytic training. To my mind this is an extraordinarily interesting experiment, demanding not only respect but also follow-up.

When it comes to high costs to an institute, see also Weiss 1982.

6. It is interesting to note that this development was perceived as early as 1946:

> It is paradoxical that there is a group that is unfit for the career of an analyst because there are too few psychoneurotic symptoms. They are well adapted to reality and, as far as any outward sign goes, well integrated, except that they show a certain rigidity due to an obvious prominence of narcissistic traits. These people have succeeded in a full repression of their psychic conflicts with the help of a powerful narcissistic defense. . . . Attempts to acquaint them with the language of the unconscious is like discussing color schemes with the blind. It is hardly necessary to add that this remoteness from their own unconscious precludes any real understanding of the unconscious of others, although they may have an intellectual grasp of its mechanisms. [H. Sachs 1947:161]

7. Concerning intuition—"physiognomic judgment"—see Bernfeld 1962:471–473.

8. Concerning the analyst's need of a personal analysis Freud had said at the Second Psychoanalytic Congress in Nürnberg in 1910 that "It seems that the pre-requisite for a successful application of psycho-analytical technique is that the physician should begin his analytical training by being analysed himself" (quoted in Kovács 1936:349). Two years later, this evolved into:

> If the doctor is to be in a position to use his unconscious in this way as an instrument in the analysis, he must himself fulfil one psycho-

logical condition to a high degree. He may not tolerate any resistances in himself which hold back from his consciousness what has been perceived by his unconscious; otherwise he would introduce into the analysis a new species of selection and distortion which would be far more detrimental than that resulting from concentration of conscious attention. It is not enough for this that he himself should be an approximately normal person. It may be insisted, rather, that he should have undergone a psycho-analytic purification and have become aware of those complexes of his own which would be apt to interfere with his grasp of what the patient tells him. There can be no reasonable doubt about the disqualifying effect of such defects in the doctor; every unresolved repression in him constitutes what has been aptly described by Stekel as a "blind spot" in his analytic perception. [Freud 1912:116]

9. Oberndorf reports that all reading of *analytica* was forbidden while applicants remained in analysis (1926:321).

10. Since the twenties and thirties the tendency has been toward more pronounced character analyses. One pioneer in this area was Wilhelm Reich, who, however, was probably on to the issue a bit too early for the psychoanalytic movement and was marginalized (but for other reasons). Another—and theoretically perhaps more refined—character analyst was Karen Horney, who, when she was threatened with losing her status as training analyst at the New York Psychoanalytic Society in 1942, left the Society and thereby also the IPA.

11. "Patients enter analysis today not with a phobia or an obsession but because they are 'nervous,' or, as one young patient recently put it, 'My problems are just in two areas, my work and with girls'" (Rangell 1974:3).

12. Freud's opinion was that the main function of training analysis is to "enable his teacher to make a judgement as to whether the candidate can be accepted for further training" (Freud 1937:248).

13. Nacht (1954:250) enumerates some points where he feels able to discern that the candidate's underlying motives for seeking analysis are diametrically opposed to those of the ordinary analysand.

14. Aarons maintains that this whole dichotomy between symptom- and character-oriented analyses is rather misleading, quoting Ernst Kris saying that "it is an illusion to think that there are any easy analytic cases" (1982–1983:684).

15. This may possibly be a valid statement only so long as psychoanalysis is a profession that is sought after (see the section "Psychoanalysis and Its Uncertain Future" in Chapter 6).

16. See also H. Sachs 1947:161.

17. For a personally revealing discussion of this topic, see Herulf 1993.

18. Of course the old way of viewing things did not vanish at once, but continued having its defenders.

19. For a review of the literature treating the issue of analyzability, see Bachrach and Leaff 1978.

20. According to Clara Thompson, at an early stage the William Alanson White Institute in New York had taken a stance against all reporting on the part of the training analyst (Thompson 1958:48). On the other hand, William Alanson White was not a component society of the IPA (and still is not).

21. For a more detailed discussion on the drawbacks of the reporting system, see Kairys 1964, Greenacre 1966, and McLaughlin 1973.

22. Responsibility was, of course, not only an issue for the candidate. Greenacre points out what difficulties a training analyst may encounter when he is to convey information as to the grounds for the rejection of an unsuitable candidate (Greenacre 1961:38). To some, the conflict has become so great that they prefer to abstain from saying anything, whereas with others there has been some kind of reconciliation with the cruelty of the task: "I have stopped feeling guilty towards my candidate when the problem of his suitability becomes actual" (Heimann 1968:533). On the handling of the problem candidate, see also McLaughlin 1973:704.

23. When it comes to those institutes that have adopted a nonreporting system, but have retained the requirement that the training analyst must inform the institute when the analysis is terminated, Hagedorn is of the opinion that an implicit bond concerning the end of the analysis is created between analyst and candidate, which in turn will become a nonanalyzable mutual secret (Hagedorn 1992:86).

24. The Swedish Psychoanalytic Society had a system where it was possible in some measure to ascertain the effects of the personal analysis without involving it in the educational process itself. This was achieved by interviewing the candidates within a two-year interval before they were accepted for training. In that way it was possible to evaluate their development under analysis (see Wallerstein 1978:494).

25. There are exceptions to this seemingly total hegemony: the IPA societies in Barcelona, Denmark, Norway, Vienna, and England (details from Cremerius 1995:11).

In the British Society the training analyst must still inform the Institute every six months as to the progress of his analysand candidates. He is also expected to give his approval when the candidate is ready to embark upon seminars, and later, as the latter commences supervised work. Finally, he is to give a statement in advance of the candidate's graduation. From what I have been able to ascertain in discussions with members of this Society, the whole procedure seems to run rather smoothly without any serious hangups. That is, of course, something that would merit an investigation of its own, but for that there is no room here. The fact that London today has the head office of the IPA and has supplanted the United States as the main theoretical center of psychoanalysis most certainly plays an important role. When the theoretical center of gravity combines with power one could expect a streak of condescension and conservatism to develop, promoting a willingness both to defend and to suffer a reporting system: "One can read into the answers given by the British informants that they were convinced the training in their institute was the best in the world, giving them the right to look down a little upon the state of affairs in institutes across the channel" (Thomä 1993:28).

26. McLaughlin (1973:699, 707) concludes that when one abolishes the reporting system and gives less weight to the training analysis the remaining institutional functions—especially the seminars and the supervised cases—are obliged to sharpen their attention to the candidates and, not in the least, the understanding of their own roles.

27. That training analyses now, for the first time, could be purely therapeutic does not solve the obvious problem that (possible) candidates often are not in analysis because of a personally felt need of therapeutic help, but because it is a basic requirement for access to training. Nielsen came up with a drastic suggestion to solve the problem of the "cool" training analyses: "The analyst's first and foremost job ought then to be to make a patient out of the analysand or, to put it in English, to make him suffer" (1954:247). But if it is correct that from the time when psychoanalysis won social acceptance and attained its status as a profession applicants and candidates have come to display an annoying "normalcy," it might be easier said than done to make the candidate suffer.

28. For a discussion on problematic identificatory processes between training analysts and candidates, see, for example, Greenacre 1966 or Hagedorn 1992.

29. It is often maintained that none of this should be displayed by a professionally neutral analyst, but of course it always is, which to my mind is part of both the charm and the harm of the whole matter. In *Reflecting Psychoanalysis* I discuss this issue on a more theoretical level in terms of a "primary symbolic structurization of the unconscious" (Reeder 1996:70–77).

30. Fleming and Weiss, too, point out that a training analysis should be expected to develop in the candidate the kind of "work ego" that Fliess speaks of: "What should be assessed is the growth and development of certain ego functions necessary for analytic competence and scholarship" (1978:42).

31. An interesting study on how the transference develops after a training analysis is presented in Norman and colleagues 1976.

32. For a comprehensive summary of what Freud has written about the setting, see Böhm 1999:496–497.

33. "The ethics of our profession can be summarized, I think, by saying that we should not exploit our patients, especially considering the vulnerability and strength of transference relationships, in any way—emotionally, behaviourally, sexually, or financially" (Coltart 1993:42).

34. In American ego psychology one has often relied upon the concept of an "average expectable environment," which designates a hypothetical "normal" milieu where the child's needs could be expected to be met to an adequate degree. Soon after I had imagined myself to have coined the expression "average expectable psychoanalyst" I discovered that it (of course) already was in existence (see Wallerstein 1981a). The difference between Wallerstein's use of the term and mine is that in his case the average analyst is understood from the point of view of the needy analysand, whereas in my case he is perceived from the vantage point of the needs and demands of the psychoanalytic community.

35. To some extent this might be ascribed to the fact that institutes with a Kleinian orientation have a greater tendency to accept candidates who are "sicker" (and therefore require longer treatments) (see Wallerstein 1978:486).

36. In an interview with Anthony Molino, Nina Coltart—who at the time stood independent from all groups within the British Society—offers one of the most candid characterizations of this movement that I have come across: "The Kleinians . . . are a religious movement, while the rest of us aren't. And fanatical religious movements believe that they possess the truth, and are prepared to impose it at practically any cost to other people. That is going on all the time in the British Society . . . under a veneer of civility which is so phony I can't tell you" (Molino 1997:172).

37. For a discussion on clinical aspects of the reanalysis, see Szalita 1968 and also Wagner 1963. For a discussion on analyzing colleagues, see Berman 1995.

38. For a description of group supervision at the Paris Psychoanalytical Society, see Israël 1992.

39. For a discussion on analysis three contra four sessions or more per week against a background of theoretical differences between different societies, see Israël 1994. See also Laufer's commentary (1994).

40. For a brief discussion on supervision problems that may be caused by the personality of the supervisor, see Grinberg 1970:378.

41. There is one exception. In the Swedish Psychoanalytical Society, anyone appointed since 1987 as a training analyst (with the authorization to analyze candidates) must undergo a two-year supervision training program before he may supervise independently. A program of that kind, as far as I have been able to discern, is unique to the Swedish Society, and we are still lacking a comprehensive literature through which it would be possible for supervisors to improve themselves (see Szecsödy 1994:126–127).

42. Haesler (1993) suggests instead that the conflict between the teacher and the analyst is the explanation for the problematic nature of the supervisory function. Haesler's way of defining the central conflict of supervision is

closer to my understanding of the field of tension between "patient-" and "therapist-oriented" supervision, which I thus see as one of the manifestations of the pedagogical conflict.

43. But: "the time is not ripe for this until his analysis has reached the point where his interest is no longer focussed on himself but genuinely on the outside world" (Kovács 1936:351).

44. It is not unusual for candidates to be asked to evaluate courses, theoretical seminars, and their teachers, either individually or in groups. Less commonly, the institute gathers any kind of corresponding information as to the candidates' experience in the supervisory situation (Martin et al. 1978). On the whole, what has been written on supervision in psychoanalytic training seems to almost exclusively have been formulated from the perspective of the institute and practically never from a candidate's perspective. See, however, Shevrin (1981a,b), who, with considerable moral integrity, writes about the subtle methods of repression that can be found in the supervisory situation.

45. For a well-balanced discussion of these problems, see Baudry 1993. For a comprehensive perspective on the different functions and difficulties inherent in supervision, plus a suggestion for their solution, see Blomfield 1985.

46. "At present there are some training analysts who believe that there should be much greater freedom to discontinue training of candidates who seem unsuited for the profession. But in actual practice this is very difficult for many to do—especially where the burden of the decision lies almost wholly with the training analyst" (Greenacre 1961:38).

47. It is not quite certain that supervised cases that are terminated "prematurely" must be judged to be failures or even as a sign of a candidate's lacking aptitude. A recently conducted investigation at Columbia University Psychoanalytic Center for Training and Research shows that in their institute 35 percent of supervised cases were terminated prematurely, which is to say before any meaningful psychoanalytic process had been inaugurated. For this reason the authors suggest that any "failed" case should be regarded as part of the training experience and not excluded as some kind of anomaly, judged against the background of otherwise "impeccable" cases (Glick et al. 1996:803).

48. For a discussion of the dynamic and structural factors underlying different forms of distortion of clinical reporting, see Spence 1997.

49. In a footnote the authors assert that "there is no reference in psychoanalytic or sociological literature to this issue" (Dulchin and Segal 1982b:34). Pollock establishes that any attention paid to the newly graduated psychoanalyst's achievements has been habitually neglected (1976:327), which could be a sign of the same thing, namely that the invisible and secret control procedures are far-reaching and give rise to a form of guilt that stimulates the impulse to do nothing at all.

50. "The senior analysts believed that in using the information acquired from patients and sharing it with colleagues in evaluating junior members, confidentiality was being sustained so long as two conditions were met: (1) the source of analytic confidences must remain anonymous; (2) the relationships between source and junior member, and between source and analyst must remain undisclosed" (Dulchin and Segal 1982b:34).

51. For a discussion on the importance of the supervisor's attention with regard to the candidate's personality or character, see Baudry 1993:604–607.

52. Completely aside from such legal issues as who carries the responsibility for the treatment, the supervisor's responsibility in his capacity as the conscience of the supervised case is a reality that neither he nor the candidate can avoid. As long as the candidate's work is satisfactory the supervisor can exercise his responsibility passively, but when he fears that the candidate's achievements are not useful or are even deleterious to the analysand things will, of course, be radically different. The mere risk of this happening may give rise to a controlling element creeping in even when it is not really called for.

Chapter 5

1. For an extensive discussion on the place and function of love in the professional encounter—and not least faith in the victory of love over hate as part of the therapeutic ideology—see Halmos 1965.

2. Economically and administratively, psychoanalytic organizations and institutes have—with few exceptions for better or for worse—stood apart from all public institutions. In this way it has been possible for them to retain full control over a training program and a business whose intrinsic goals are very difficult to encompass by welfare institutions with their utilitarian demand for equality and what is best for all. Ideologically, psychoanalysis does tend to stand beside the ideological orientation of the welfare society (although not necessarily in opposition to it) and has had to safeguard its independence: "In relation to the surrounding world the tendency has been to close off and thereby lose realistic contact with public institutions and trends" (Beland 1983:53). See also Slavin 1997.

3. For more on the isolation of the analyst, see Greben 1975. See also King 1983:187.

4. See also Marmor 1953; Wheelis 1956; Grinberg 1963; Gitelson 1963; Wallerstein 1981a; Greben 1975, 1982–1983; Cooper 1986; Eisold 1994. For a popular and amusing/anxiety-provoking sketch of the mental problems of the professional helper, see Epstein 1997.

5. Still, the selection of training analysts remains poorly elucidated. Kairys writes that he cannot find any literature on the subject (1964:493). And as late

as 1982–1983 Dorn published an article with the title "Training Analyst Selection: The Need for Criteria."

6. See note 41 to Chapter 4.

7. In a communication by fax on March 13, 2000, with Joanne Campbell, Membership Secretary of the IPA, I was informed that of a total of 10,152 members of the IPA, 6,553 were "full members" and 3,599 "associate members." Within that same total there were 2,620 training analysts. (In 1920 the total membership of the IPA was 240 persons; 1930, 430; 1940, 450; 1950, 800; 1960, 1,515; 1970, 2,450; 1980, 5,004; 1990, 7,182; 2000, 10,100 [International Psychoanalysis: The Newsletter of the IPA 9/1:16].) "Full members" and "associate members" are all regarded as independent psychoanalysts, but for "full membership" it is often required to give a paper in one's society, demonstrating the author's clinical and/or theoretical skill and knowledge. The distinction does not exist in all IPA societies.

8. For more on feelings of bitterness and being a failure when not appointed to be a training analyst, see also Eissler 1969:469; Joseph 1983:18.

9. In the United States, the formation of convoys can be explained in many instances by how new institutes and societies have been formed. Arlow (1972) writes that when it was difficult to convince a larger group of analysts to set up a new analytic society in some specified location it was not uncommon that one or two analysts (who could be a married couple) moved to the new scene and there gradually created a group around themselves. The convoy system is no isolated American phenomenon, however. In England, from the thirties and forties until the seventies, the Kleinian movement must be said to have been a convoy system. Another well-known example is the group of analysands and supervisees who followed Jacques Lacan when he divorced himself from the French Society in 1953, a move that in the sixties gave rise to a new French organization, and during the nineties to a new psychoanalytic international (see Etchegoyen and Miller 1996).

10. Balint (1948, 1954) warns against a clinical praxis (he most probably has Kleinian analyses in mind) in which premature "deep" interpretations lead to the full emotional impact of the negative transference never being allowed to develop properly.

11. Ödman describes the immanent pedagogy as "all the forms of hidden pedagogy that permeate our lives. It is, then, a question of a pedagogy immanent in the situation itself, which seldom or never is made conscious as an influence" (Ödman 1995:x).

12. The question of whether ego ideal and superego should be kept apart or if it is best to stick to Freud's model has been a subject of debate ever since he introduced the superego concept. For a short survey, see, for example, Sandler 1960; Sandler, Holder, and Meers 1963. In a well-known article from 1960, "The Loving and Beloved Superego in Freud's Structural Theory,"

Schafer makes an attempt to put right what he sees as a skewed conception of the superego, making of it merely or mainly a condemning and judging instance. He is seeking that function whereby we may also love and respect ourselves—that is, keep up our self-regard. To my mind, however, Schafer's effort to evoke a loving and beloved superego only results in his reducing the superego to an abstraction comprising the subject's evaluations of itself, positive and negative. To put the matter slightly differently: he abandons any possible conception of the superego as a phenomenologically discernible mental instance. The voice of the superego comes from the outside, as it were, as an alien presence, no matter how familiar it may be to the subject. The same can scarcely be said of the ego's consoling, inciting, and praising functions. The discrepancy between these two instances explains why Freud never managed to arrive at any deeper understanding of a "loving and beloved superego"— his interest is totally directed toward the condemning and pursuing superego.

13. Freud's way of developing his concept of a death drive might possibly satisfy the mythological need for a pristine matrix of human aggressivity, man's destructiveness, and life's inexorable itinerary toward its own extinction (which in fact is the same as the drive's attraction to the state that prevailed before life itself). But to gather both psychological and biological phenomena under the same roof like that makes the concept itself so exceedingly speculative that it loses all credibility; it simply fits very badly with the phenomenology of inner experience. The more the proponents of this idea exert themselves in their attempts to convey a sense of credibility, the less they seem to convince.

When it comes to the hate under discussion here, I will leave unsaid whether it should be viewed primarily as a derivate of the drives or as a result of the subject's interaction with its environment.

14. In my book, *Reflecting Psychoanalysis*, I devote a lengthier discussion to the phenomenon of hate than can be afforded here (Reeder 1996:159–174).

15. When it comes to the tendency for primitive psychic processes to develop within larger groups, see Kernberg 1986:823.

16. It is not often that one sees hate mentioned as a dynamic factor in the inner life of organizations. Offhand I can only recall how the communist movement once used to make something desirable out of something ugly by idealizing what was called "class hatred." That hate does permeate society should come as no surprise to anyone considering the historical facts, but it seems as if we have only had the courage to call a spade a spade as long as it was possible to forge hate into something heroic. As a counterbalance to such measures, the welfare society has been the brave attempt of modernity to neutralize hate, although very seldom addressing the true affective issues, resulting instead in a tendency to idealize envy (or at least give it ideological/political support).

17. In his book, *Attention and Interpretation*, Bion (1970) discusses, with the help of an allegory of sorts, the relationship between what he calls "the mystic" and "the establishment," which in many respects touches upon our hypothesis concerning an analytical superego complex. It is interesting to note that in the analytic literature there are few reactions to this perhaps most vehement of commentaries concerning life within analytic institutions (see, however, Langs 1978 or Rustin 1985).

18. Dulchin and Segal write: "A student who recommended an analyst of the Institute to a relative or friend might be setting up a channel for the flow of information which could ultimately endanger his career" (1982b:31). Apparently, the problem does not concern only candidates, but the system as a whole.

19. Cf.: "The much lambasted tendency of psychoanalysts to accuse their adversaries of being defensive and one another of being 'insufficiently analysed' is not some accident or lamentable falling from the high standards of the psychoanalytic enterprise. It is *structured into* psychoanalysis, because there is no way that one can be sure that this claim (of resistance, for example) can be wrong" (Frosch 1998:15–16, italics in original).

20. On the tendency to orthodoxy and the evolution of cliques based upon strong identificatory processes among psychoanalysts, see Eisold 1997. On the need among psychoanalysts to establish groups around a strong leader and how that began with Freud, see Roustang 1976. For a history of breaks, splits, and the struggle for psychoanalytic authority within the New York Psychoanalytical Society during the forties, see Eisold 1998. For a similar history of the wrenching controversy between Kleinians and Anna Freudians during the same period, see Steiner 1985.

21. Those analysts who themselves had suffered the same difficulties and anguish as their analysands come to mind. Although often sensitive, gifted, and theoretically precise, they have been marginalized with considerable precision throughout the history of the psychoanalytic movement. The rest—the "normal" ones—have kept to their excluding stance: disregard the analysand's reality, expel "deviant" colleagues. Bonomi (1999) gives a good picture of how the stamp of insanity could be employed to discredit Freud's once perhaps most cherished pupil, Sándor Ferenczi.

22. For a detailed picture of the dynamics in the relations between colleagues in psychoanalytic societies and institutes, see Grinberg 1963.

23. For a discussion of the reluctance of psychoanalysts to reveal too much about themselves for fear that it might have repercussions upon their standing among colleagues, see Kantrowitz 1999. In this article the author also discusses the analytic myth of normality.

24. Ten years later Thomä comments that Sandler inadvertently here might have demonstrated what an unwelcome effect the training system might have on psychoanalytic practice (1993:37).

25. Balint notes that the goals of the Berlin Institute included "therapy for the broad masses, research and training. In fact what they—and all other institutes—have achieved is only a system of training" (1948:168). As to research itself, he writes that the results have been so meager that they scarcely deserve mention.

Research and/or theoretical collaboration with other disciplines has never been a matter of course in the history of the psychoanalytic movement. Not that there has been no cooperation with other disciplines, but it has most often been a case of psychoanalysis being the generous and willing donor of ideas to the development of some other system of knowledge. Psychoanalysis has remained a relatively closed system of knowledge and analytical publications show few references to forms of knowing other than the analytic ones (Holzman 1976). In his fictitious directions for an imperious institute Kernberg writes: "Avoid accepting and training the maverick who wishes to learn psychoanalysis to apply it to another realm of professional endeavour, the philosopher interested in the boundaries between philosophical and psychoanalytic understanding, the empirical researcher wishing to complement his neuropsychological background" (1996:1038). Sometimes an analyst with a previous background in academic research either has abandoned these interests and become an analyst like everyone else, or carried on his research while maintaining an absolute division between this and his analytic activities (see Thomä 1993:8). Those who relegate clinical work to the background and instead devote themselves to applied psychoanalysis and research have been treated with condescension by the general body of psychoanalysts and have been allotted to second rank among their colleagues (see Ferber and Krent 1976:448). The problem is not a lack of academicians, but the inability to leave room for an intellectually open and honest scientific discussion.

These conditions do, however, seem to be changing. Due to essential initiatives taken by the central offices within the IPA during the nineties, especially with the formation of the Committee on Psychoanalytic Research in 1990, empirical research has gained acceptance and has hit its stride. This may very well be due to the above-mentioned fact that empirical research has been lacking a tradition of its own within psychoanalysis. Therefore it does not pose any substantial threat to any established institutional structures (which does not preclude that it might very well threaten established conceptions concerning the nature of the psychoanalytic enterprise).

For a comprehensive history of the IPA's and the APA's treatment of the research issue, see Wallerstein and Fonagy 1999 (also Wallerstein 1978). For a deeper presentation of the present status of research within psychoanalysis, see Shapiro and Emde 1995 (also Thomä 1993:6–16).

26. Such a way of viewing things often combines smoothly with a tendency to emphasize the scientific nature of psychoanalysis.

27. For a more extensive discussion of the arrogance of Knowledge, see Reeder 1996:18–20.

28. Freud's position was that the only worldview proper to psychoanalysis would be the scientific one, asserting that "there are no sources of knowledge of the universe other than the intellectual working-over of carefully scrutinized observations" (Freud 1933:159). I can agree with the last statement concerning observations as long as one adds to it "carefully retrieved experience."

29. For quotation source see http://eseries.ipa.org.uk/prev/newsletter/97-1/rangell.htm Rangell's worries concerning the theoretical diversification within psychoanalysis go back a long time; see Rangell 1982, 1988. For a historical survey of the tendency of psychoanalysis to theoretical diversification, see Bergmann 1993. For an impassioned defense of theoretical pluralism, see Feyerabend 1975.

30. Guttman has a very creative suggestion for criteria for what might be viewed as "deviant" within psychoanalytic discourse: "Deviant theories . . . are theories formulated by men and women whose aspiration it is to create a scientific revolution, but whose creative powers fall short of their aspirations" (1985:169). Just like Icarus, the deviant swerves too high; his fall does not depend upon his wish to fly, but upon a lacking sense of judgment or good navigation. Anyone who really wishes to establish a "scientific revolution"—in the way, for example, that Freud did—is no deviant, even if he might have begun his career as a psychoanalyst; he is a *founder* (and, it is hoped, as Guttman intimates, the founder has the good judgment to call his invention something other than "psychoanalysis"). The others will remain deviants because they have been unsuccessful in leaving the very model that they might most have wished to abandon.

Ergo: Anyone striving to better analytic knowing—whatever the result—is never a deviant.

31. Britton also writes: "Small distortions, totemic use of terms, detours into irrelevant references, links made with other work not clearly connected to the thesis; all are prompted by our desire for affiliation and our fear of exile" (1994:1222). He continues by saying that in our day whenever more analysts move between differing subgroups ("schools") and at the same time uncertainty prevails over whether psychoanalytic theory is about to disintegrate or if it will stride toward integration, publication anxiety may be expected to grow and with that the continued distortion of others' texts.

32. Despite close to fifty percent of those selected for psychoanalytic training being women, their representation within the centers of power is far from proportional to their number. Cremerius has observed that of all IPA presidents only one—Phyllis Greenacre—has been a woman. In Germany only 25 percent of training analysts are women.

33. In Langs's article from 1978 there is an account of how a text by Harold Searles, written when he himself was a candidate at the end of the forties in the United States, was refused and subsequently left untouched in a drawer. This article addressed many of the issues concerning countertransference that were to surface in England just a couple of years later and have become so central to the evolution of the clinical practice of psychoanalysis.

34. If one reads Stout 1993, it will be abundantly clear that the expected ethos surely does not come about by itself.

35. See Olinick et al. 1973:145. For a deeper discussion on the significance of the Hippocratic oath for the psychoanalytic attitude, see McLaughlin 1961.

36. An official professional psychoanalytic ethic of the kind one finds within other professions has long been missing. In 1998, however, the Executive Council of the IPA confirmed an ethical set of rules for its component societies. In part, this late arrival may be ascribed to the fact that the occupational groups most often eligible for psychoanalytic training—mostly physicians and psychologists—are relying upon an ethical code already in their original occupation.

37. McLaughlin interprets the physician's readiness to work at least in part as a response to the opinion of society that he should really not gain any (moral or personal) satisfaction, something that is conveyed with the tacit attitude that "the only good doctor is the one busy to the point of exhaustion" (1961:116).

38. For a candid description of what the work schedule of a doctor analyst may look like, see Kelman 1970. By way of identification, Freud's capacity for work has influenced generations of psychoanalysts; for an illustration of his views concerning work and of his actual work schedule, see Riesman 1950.

39. Wellendorf has pointed out something that seldom appears in the discussions, namely that there can be serious consequences if the impact of psychoanalytic training both on physicians and on those with a background in academic psychology is not negotiated and worked through (1995:146). To both these groups, all previous knowledge is so estranged from what they encounter in the psychoanalytic experience that they are faced with a loyalty conflict: What may there really be of value in what I have done up until now? The psychoanalyst in many ways has shifted from one culture to another, and whether this conflict is solved by eschewing previous knowledge and convictions or by embedding psychoanalysis in suppressed suspicion and reservation, the damage takes place as the analyst is divided, weakening his work ego and tempting him to sabotage the integrity of the analytic treatment. "The process of socialization required for one to become a psychoanalyst . . . must be understood as a *resocialization* where both primary and secondary socializations undergo transformation. The model for such transformation is religious conversion" (Beland 1983:43, italics in original). This aspect of the acquisition of an identity as psy-

choanalyst has been neglected most probably due to a pervasive desire to perceive psychoanalysis as a branch of medicine and/or general psychology. To a considerably greater extent, the critical transition from an established identity as a psychotherapist to that of a psychoanalyst has been discussed during the seventies and the eighties (see Joseph and Wallerstein 1982).

40. See Rosenbloom 1992 for a closer depiction of the first period after matriculation. In passing, it may be pointed out that Rosenbloom relies on a conception of the psychoanalyst's superego as a prescriptive instance (p. 118).

41. "Idealization as a stage in psychoanalytic theory development and in learning psychoanalytic theory is . . . virtually universal, in part because of an exaggerated and incorrect distinction between theory and practice built almost inevitably into analytic education" (Fogel and Glick 1991:414).

The ways of addressing the issue of idealization as mentioned here are manifold. Rothstein (1980), for example, writes of the analyst's narcissistic investment in his theory of choice, whereas Rangell (1982) speaks of "transference to theory." On the sense of superiority that can arise from idealizations, see Marmor 1953.

42. For references concerning the emotional stress that can afflict the analyst in his professional function, see note 4 to this chapter.

43. See also Gitelson 1962a:195; Thomä 1993:33.

44. "Graduation from an institute represents a potential time of fulfillment and rite of passage, symbolically and experientially. . . . Oftentimes, however, initial joy and excitement are followed by profound feelings of depression" (Dorn 1982–1983:697).

45. See Thickstun 1985:195.

46. See also Grinberg 1989.

47. Cf.: "I am personally of the opinion that a necessary condition for the training of the psychoanalyst is to allow him to speak about the difficulty of his task, and that we should, with him, evaluate these difficulties. But this implies that the debate must be left open within our institutions, and that our difficulties remain a subject for communication" (Widlöcher 1983:33). On the critical period after matriculation and the importance of societies and institutes catering to this problem, see Kestemberg 1978:506.

48. For a summary of Fenichel's reasoning, see Reich 1941. Yet another reason for cherishing the superego is that many of us can experience its attacks as a welcome "cleansing" of the soul—as if by regularly subjecting oneself to its wrath one were paying for one's right to life.

49. Despite its apparent relevance, the newly graduated analyst's age is seldomly discussed, something that of course is connected to the age at which he is accepted for training: "In many respects we are out of sync with the developmental life cycle" (Buechler 1988:466). Age is most often positively correlated with what we like to refer to as maturity. An older analyst is expected

to possess more wisdom than a younger one, but we may well ask ourselves if this compensates to an acceptable degree for the shorter time he has at his disposal after graduation to free himself from the professional superego he in all probability has acquired. Isn't it perhaps rather that when a candidate of more advanced age graduates, he runs the risk of becoming an analyst who will remain under the rule of his superego, whereas a younger candidate may become an analyst with more time on his hands to come to grips with the destructive effects of the analytic institution?

50. For more concerning the effects of psychotherapy upon psychoanalytic training, see Joseph and Wallerstein 1982.

51. For a thorough discussion on the restraining effects of theory (especially theory of technique) on the analytic dialogue, see Arlow 1995. See also Ogden 1996.

52. The matter is in part founded in the training analyst institution's need to avoid observation from outside: "The training analyst's 'going into hiding' on the professional level . . . operates in unconscious collusion with the candidate's assumption that it is the training analyst 'who knows' about the candidate's unconscious, rather than the candidate who is himself finding out about his unconscious with the help of the training analyst" (Kernberg 1986:817).

53. Cf. also, "The idea that the patient has to fight against a sort of 'enemy within' seems to have influenced some psychoanalysts to see their work with their patients as a sort of battle in which the analyst has to fight with the enemy in the patient" (Sandler and Dreher 1996:14).

54. Cf.:

> Just as everything the patient feels about his analyst is called "transference," there is a converse tendency to call everything the analyst feels about his patient "countertransference." The result is excessive emphasis on the concept of projective identification, which is thereby to some extent abused. To base all interpretations on countertransference feelings that are exclusively a consequence of projective identification is to deny what the patient has to say. The theory of the countertransference has little by little become a defence against the impact of the reality of the analytic relationship— a defence which belongs to the analyst and not to the patient. [Treurniet 1993:877; see also Limentani 1986:239; on projective identification, see Ogden 1979]

55. Touching upon the same issue, Arlow paraphrases Freud: "Where superego was, there shall ego be" (1989:165).

56. The notion of the psychoanalyst's inner career was born in discussions at the beginning of the eighties with Dr. Tony Sporrong in Färjestaden, Sweden.

57. A survey of the issues confronting the newly matriculated analyst can be found in Schafer 1979. The best that I can think of in this genre, which really picks up what is truly personal, are Goldberg 1992 and Gerson 1996. There are excellent studies that chart the analyst's or the therapist's professional development, but mainly on the descriptive level, which really does not capture the inner and very subjective process underlying observable changes: good examples are Stoltenberg and Delworth 1987, or Skovholt and Rønnestad 1992. For an interesting theoretical exposé of the development from knowledge to competence, see the chapter "Five Steps from Novice to Expert" in Dreyfus and Dreyfus 1986.

58. See also Isakower 1939; Alexander 1925:27.

59. For a more extensive discussion on the function of the narratheme in the subject's reflection and narrating, see Reeder 1996, Chapter 4.

60. When the empirical ego fails to live up to the demands of the ideal, the superego will easily be activated. Then there must be sufficient room for withstanding its eroding effects and for sustaining love of the self.

61. "Like all learning procedures, one starts with a set of rules, then learns to violate the rules for virtuoso purposes" (Levenson 1982:12). For a description of how a group of recently graduated analysts worked with texts of Freud to transform knowledge into competence, see Fogel and Glick 1991. For a description of one analyst's work coping with the "orthodox" American ego psychology and finding a theoretical alternative, see Slap 1996.

62. Cf.: "Supervision . . . prolongs a dependent student status, creates multiple identifications, and delays finding an independent, personal style" (Bak 1970:19). To continually look throughout one's career for every opportunity to get new supervision is illustrative of the power of the professional superego. It may seem as if personal development is striven for, but in fact one is always welcoming the opportunity of having one's professional superego both reinforced and confirmed. The supervisor, and sometimes also the other members of a supervisory group, allow the superego to manifest itself in the shape of real persons to be idealized and/or feared.

Chapter 6

1. See also Cremerius 1986, 1987 and Thomä 1993.

2. However urgent the task may be, it is beyond the scope of this survey to analyze or estimate in any deeper sense the possible political intentions within the psychoanalytic movement of today.

3. In addition, the obvious need for the "analyst's analyst" (i.e., an experienced analyst who shares the fundamental values of the institute, but stands outside of its administrative functions) could in this way be met. Since he has no influence whatsoever upon the careers of other analysts, a psychoanalyst

in need of help may safely turn to such a person with confidence that total confidentiality will be upheld.

4. Aarons writes: "We cannot contend that a training analysis is or should be more thorough than an nontraining analysis. . . . In the present context, 'more or less analysis' is meaningless. . . . Is the analysand analyzable or not, and can the analyst analyze him if he is analyzable? When it comes down to this formulation," what difference is permissible between a training and a nontraining analyst?" (1982–1983:683).

5. Thomä suggests that one limit the minimal requirements for a personal analysis to somewhere between three and four hundred sessions, but with a retained high frequency (of three to five sessions per week) (1993:56, 59–60). In Thomä and Kächele (1999:34), this demand has been reduced to two hundred sessions.

6. At least part of the inspiration for this model has, in all probability, come from Jacques Lacan's Freudian School in Paris, where one tried to uphold the idea that "only the analyst can authorize himself." In other words, this is a notion of the psychoanalyst that very much coincides with the rule for any analyst during the first epoch.

During the seventies Lacan made an attempt at theorizing this whole matter by maintaining the idea that a complete analysis would end in the analysand himself becoming an analyst. At the same time, in 1967, he had put forth his *Proposition*, a document that gave rise to violent repercussions and splits within the Lacanian movement (Lacan 1978). Here he suggests a procedure that was to be called *la passe*—"the passage"—where one who is at the end of his personal analysis relays, through two mediators ("*passeurs*"—most often other analysands who have not yet reached this point in their own analyses), before a committee of elected analysts the story of the significant turning point in his own analysis. If his narrative is accepted as valid, he will be awarded the title *Analyste de l'école*, which makes him a member of the highest caste. Of course, *la passe* soon turned out to become the Lacanian equivalent to the institutions of the training analyst and the training analysis as previously known within the IPA. In fact, this example demonstrates to what high degree claims for power do permeate the psychoanalytic movement, even when it tries to rid itself of its very own power games. *La passe* also turned out to be a great fiasco—during the seventies and eighties very few dared or could undergo the trial, and tragedies ensued when some of these could not "pass."

7. For an interesting description of a deliberate attempt to conduct training in psychotherapy under explicitly nonauthoritarian conditions, see Lomas 1990.

8. In December 1998, the Executive Committee of the IPA approved the formation of the Committee on Psychoanalytic Education (COMPSED), the tasks of which were enumerated as:

1. Developing methods for investigating how different forms of psycho-analytic training may give rise to differing ways of conducting psychoanalytic practice.
2. Delimiting relevant training variables and judging how these may affect instructors and candidates.
3. Making an estimate of the extent to which relevant training variables accord with existing goals and with the institute's general philosophy of training.
4. Including in methodological development direct contacts between members of COMPSED and all who are engaged in the training programs of the studied institutes, just like those partaking in clinical activities and discussions.
5. Supporting fresh initiative within psychoanalytic training with an aim to strengthen psychoanalytic institutes when it comes to effectively establishing and promulgating fresh knowledge to new generations of psychoanalysts.

9. In a survey conducted during the seventies, Knowles discovered that adult students prefer self-direction; the experience of adults is a rich source of further learning, and they will learn better and more quickly by discussions and problem solving rather than by passive listening. The learning of adults is based upon competence, which is to say that they wish to develop a certain degree of competence or attain a circumscribed amount of knowledge that they can then apply pragmatically in their immediate reality (Knowles 1973; for a summary of Knowles's argument, see also Zemke and Zemke 1995; for some thoughts specifically touching upon the training of adults in analytic institutes, see Szasz 1958:606–607).

10. See Wallerstein 1978:484 on England and France in this respect. Adam Phillips suggests that candidates in training should be allowed to study the literature of their own choice (quoted in Molino 1997:142).

11. The second important place for such transmission is, of course, analytic work under supervision.

12. I will not delve here into what in the Anglo-Saxon world has become known as "Psychoanalytic Studies," a kind of education in psychoanalytic ideas most often devoid of clinical exposure or training, which can be found in the United States and England (see Stanton and Reason 1996). For a definition of "Psychoanalytic Studies," see Hall 1996:71–72.

13. See note 8 to this chapter and note 25 to Chapter 5.

14. Not least is this development an effect of the theoretical self-examination undertaken by American psychoanalysis starting at the end of the sixties and the beginning of the seventies, and to a large extent brought about by a growing distrust of three decades of ego psychology attempting to compile

an encyclopedically encompassing metapsychology. For a discussion of the
new theoretical diversification, which has in many ways set the agenda for
several of the subsequent major discussions on this issue, see Wallerstein
1988. The state of contemporary psychoanalysis in this respect is well depicted
by D. M. Sachs:

> Some analysts believe it is sufficient to analyse the oedipal conflicts
> thoroughly, while others believe these must be reduced to pre-oedi-
> pal issues; some analysts require the patient to be in possession of a
> detailed biography of his development, while others are content if
> the biography is incomplete as long as symptoms are understood and
> the method for learning more is transmitted to the analysand; some
> analysts place more emphasis on sexual conflicts as primary and
> analyse aggression as a derivative, while others stress aggression as a
> separate primary motivating force; etc. [1992:147]

15. How this may come to the fore in the individual analyst is succinctly
captured by Roudinesco as she writes that

> the psychoanalysts of today . . . are nearer than their predecessors to
> the social deprivation they have to confront in their work. They are
> more pragmatic, simpler, more humanistic and more alive to all forms
> of mental suffering, even if they are sometimes less cultured than
> earlier generations of psychoanalysts. Finally, they are more unpreju-
> diced about all forms of therapy, as if declining to be imprisoned in
> dogma or sectarianism. [1997, http://eseries.ipa.org.uk/prev/newslet-
> ter/97-1/roudin.htm.

16. During the first two decades of the twentieth century Vienna was the
psychoanalytic center. During the twenties competition became more prominent as the Berlin Institute was established and rapidly became a model for
the organization of clinics and analytic training. During the thirties American
psychoanalysis began showing evidence of its power. But up until Freud's
death and World War II the psychoanalytic movement remained in all essential aspects homogeneous. Freud's presence had guaranteed the existence of
an authoritative interpretation of the meaning of psychoanalysis (for a description of Freud's strategies in developing such an interpretation, see Winter 1999).
With Freud's death all this changed rapidly, and after the war the United States
came to form the new center of psychoanalysis—theoretically and clinically
with the so-called ego psychology, institutionally with the strong ties of psychoanalysis with psychiatry and the medical establishment.

Since the latter part of the thirties, as the only really heavyweight contender
for hegemony, the British Psychoanalytical Society has held the function of host
organization for the IPA, and by dint of that shared places at the center together

with the Americans. With prominent names such as Jones, Klein, Balint and Winnicott, the English psychoanalysts had been developing a theoretical tradition of their own, albeit a diversified one, since the twenties and thirties. Here belongs, of course, Freud's daughter Anna, though her theoretical orientation turned out to be different from the other two British "schools," and in fact after the war she established rather strong ties with American ego psychology. Interestingly enough, British psychoanalysis was never a beacon for the rest of the European societies during the first two or three postwar decades. In countries like Germany or Sweden, ego psychology ruled unchallenged, while France in many ways followed its very own inclinations.

Today, the British analytical tradition must be said to have the leading role, clinically and theoretically, and this dominance has a different face in different parts of the world. In Europe, for example, the so-called object relations theory (the tradition via Balint and Winnicott) has predominated, having been developed in part as a counterweight to the Kleinian doctrine. At the same time it is frequently spiked with choice elements from her theory. In South America and Spain, Kleinian influence has been quite prominent for some time, while in North America object relations theory has been more influential in attempts to keep ego psychology alive with different attempts to integrate new theories (despite this, American psychoanalysis does remain a rather conservative bastion; see Schafer 1997b).

I would guess that the evolution of a center like the British one answers to a demand, albeit a tacit one, for stability in a time marked by great change and much uncertainty as to the future of psychoanalysis. However understandable such a request might be, it does remain a source of inertia when what is really needed is agility (see also note 25 to Chapter 4).

17. The authors were: Arlow and Brenner 1988; Michels 1988; Rangell 1988; Spruiell 1989; Reiser 1989; Wallerstein and Weinshel 1989; Orgel 1990; Cooper 1990; Richards 1990. The nine articles were subsequently summarized and commented on by Kernberg (1993).

18. The events after the death of Jacques Lacan in 1981 are illustrative of what processes may take place when a central authority suddenly is absent. Within just a couple of years there were at least twenty competing Lacanian groups. Despite the founding of a Lacanian international, the image of general division still remains (see Roudinesco 1993). One day Thomä's vision might come true: "I plead for a change of the structure and function of the IPA. It should be transformed into a predominantly scientific society. Such a reform would make it feasible to turn the administrative office of the IPA, 'Broomhills' in London, into an institute for psychoanalytic research" (Thomä 1993:12).

19. It cannot be totally ruled out that the historical role and importance of psychoanalysis for late modernity may be waning: "I think we really

shouldn't be interested in preserving psychoanalysis at all. I think that we should be interested in finding languages for what matters most to us. So far, for some people, psychoanalysis is one of these languages. It doesn't have to be. . . . I don't think psychoanalysis is there to be protected. It's there to be used and then dispensed with when something better comes along" (Phillips, quoted in Molino 1997:156–157).

References

Wherever an English edition is mentioned in the list below, quotations will be taken from that edition. In all other cases the translations are my own from the original language. *The Standard Edition of the Complete Psychological Works of Sigmund Freud* is abbreviated *S.E.*

Aarons, Z. A. (1982–1983). The training analyst concept: a superego problem. *International Journal of Psychoanalytic Psychotherapy* 9:679–689.

Alexander, F. (1925). A metapsychological description of the process of cure. *International Journal of Psycho-Analysis* 6:13–34.

APA (American Psychoanalytic Association). (1956). Minimal standards for the training of physicians in psychoanalysis. *Journal of the American Psychoanalytic Association* 4:714–721.

Arendt, H. (1958). *The Human Condition.* Chicago: University of Chicago Press, 1998.

Arlow, J. A. (1963). The supervisory situation. *Journal of the American Psychoanalytic Association* 11:576–594.

——— (1970). *Group Psychology and the Study of Institutes.* Report, Board of Professional Standards, Annual Meeting. American Psychiatric Association, San Francisco. Unpublished manuscript.

——— (1972). Some dilemmas in psychoanalytic education. *Journal of the American Psychoanalytic Association* 20:556–566.

——— (1982). Psychoanalytic education: a psychoanalytic perspective. *Annals of Psychoanalysis* X:5–20.

——— (1989). The quest for morality. In *The Psychoanalytic Core: Essays in Honor of Leo Rangell, M.D.*, ed. H. P. Blum, E. M. Weinshel, and F. R. Rodman. Madison, CT: International Universities Press.

————— (1995). Stilted listening: psychoanalysis as discourse. *Psychoanalytic Quarterly* 64:215–233.

Arlow, J. A., and Brenner, C. (1988). The future of psychoanalysis. *Psychoanalytic Quarterly* 57:1–14.

Bachrach, H. M., and Leaff, L. A. (1978). Analyzability: a systematic review of the clinical and quantitative literature. *Journal of the American Psychoanalytic Association* 26:881–920.

Bak, R. C. (1970). Psychoanalysis today. *Journal of the American Psychoanalytic Association* 18:3–23.

Baker, R. (1993). Some reflections on humour in psychoanalysis. *International Journal of Psycho-Analysis* 74:951–960.

Balint, M. (1948). On the psychoanalytic training system. *International Journal of Psycho-Analysis* 29:163–173.

————— (1954). Analytic training and training analysis. *International Journal of Psycho-Analysis* 33:157–162.

Baudry, F. D. (1993). The personal dimension and management of the supervisory situation with a special note on the parallel process. *Psychoanalytic Quarterly* 62:588–614.

Beland, H. (1983). Was ist und wozu ensteht psychoanalytische Identität? *Jahrbuch für Psychoanalyse* 15:36–67.

Benedek, T. (1954). Countertransference in the training analyst. *Bulletin of the Menninger Clinic* 18:12–16.

Berger, P. L. (1965). Towards a sociological understanding of psychoanalysis. *Social Research* 32:26–41.

Bergmann, M. S. (1993). Reflections on the history of psychoanalysis. *Journal of the American Psychoanalytic Association* 41:929–955.

————— (1997). The historical roots of psychoanalytic orthodoxy. *International Journal of Psycho-Analysis* 78:69–86.

Berman, E. (1985). Incestuous elements in psychoanalytic training. *International Psychoanalytic Studies Organization Bulletin* 7:9–10.

————— (1995). On analyzing colleagues. *Contemporary Psychoanalysis* 31:523–539.

————— (2000). Psychoanalytic supervision: the intersubjective development. *International Journal of Psycho-Analysis* 81:273–290.

Bernardi, R., and Nieto, M. (1992). What makes the training analysis "good enough?" *International Review of Psycho-Analysis* 19:137–145.

Bernfeld, S. (1962). On psychoanalytic training. *Psychoanalytic Quarterly* 31:453–482.

Bibring, E. (1937). Report of the International Training Commission. *International Journal of Psycho-Analysis* 18:365–372.

———— (1938). Report of the International Training Commission. *International Journal of Psycho-Analysis* 19:271–275.

Bibring, G. (1954). The training analysis and its place in psychoanalytic training. *International Journal of Psycho-Analysis* 53:169–173.

Bion, W. R. (1958). On hallucination. In *Second Thoughts: Selected Papers on Psycho-Analysis*. New York: Jason Aronson, 1967.

———— (1961). *Experiences in Groups and Other Papers*. London: Tavistock, 1968.

———— (1967). Notes on memory and desire. In *Classics in Psychoanalytic Technique*, ed. R. Langs. New York: Jason Aronson, 1981.

———— (1970). *Attention and Interpretation*. London: Tavistock.

———— (1997). The grid, 1963. In *Taming Wild Thoughts*. London: Karnac.

Bird, B. (1968). On candidate selection and its relation to analysis. *International Journal of Psycho-Analysis* 49:513–526.

Blitzsten, N. L., and Fleming, J. (1953). What is a supervisory psychoanalysis? *Bulletin of the Menninger Clinic* 17:117–129.

Blomfield, O. (1982). Interpretation—some general aspects. *International Review of Psycho-Analysis* 9:287–301.

———— (1985). Psychoanalytic supervision—an overview. *International Review of Psycho-Analysis* 12:401–410.

Blum, H. P. (1981). The forbidden quest and the analytical ideal: the superego and insight. *Psychoanalytic Quarterly* 50:535–556.

Bonomi, C. (1999). Flight into sanity: Jones's allegation of Ferenczi's mental deterioration reconsidered. *International Journal of Psycho-Analysis* 80:507–542.

Bourdieu, P. (1984). *Homo Academicus*. Stockholm/Stehag: Brutus Östlings förlag Symposion, 1996.

Brenner, C. (1996). The nature of knowledge and the limits of authority in psychoanalysis. *Psychoanalytic Quarterly* 65:21–31.

Britton, R. (1994). Publication anxiety: conflict between communication and affiliation. *International Journal of Psycho-Analysis* 75:1213–1224.

Britton, R. (1997). Making the private public. In *The Presentation of Case Material in Clinical Discourse*, ed. I. Ward. London: Freud Museum.

Brook, A. (1992). Psychoanalysis and commonsense psychology. *Annual of Psychoanalysis* 20:273–301.

Bruzzone, M., Casaula, E., Jimenez, J. P., and Jordan, J. F. (1985). Regression and persecution in analytic training: reflections on experience. *International Review of Psycho-Analysis* 12:411–415.

Buechler, S. (1988). Joining the psychoanalytic culture. *Contemporary Psychoanalysis* 24:462–470.

———— (1992). Stress in the personal and professional development of a psychoanalyst. *Journal of the American Academy of Psychoanalysis* 20:183–191.

Böhm, T. (1999). The difficult freedom from a plan. *International Journal of Psycho-Analysis* 80:493–505.

Calef, V. (1972). A report of the 4th pre-congress on training, Vienna 1971, to the 27th International Psycho-Analytical Congress. *International Journal of Psycho-Analysis* 53:37–45.

Calef, V., and Weinshel, E. (1973). Reporting, nonreporting, and assessment in the training analysis. *Journal of the American Psychoanalytic Association* 21:714–725.

———— (1980). The analyst as the conscience of the analysis. *International Review of Psycho-Analysis* 7:279–290.

C.E.A. (1978). Report of the study commission on the evaluation of applicants for psychoanalytic training: 143rd Bulletin of the IPA. *International Journal of Psycho-Analysis* 59:79–85.

Coltart, N. (1993). *How to Survive as a Psychotherapist*. London: Sheldon, 1996.

Cooper, A. (1984). Psychoanalysis at one hundred: beginnings of maturity. *Journal of the American Psychoanalytic Association* 31:245–267.

———— (1986). Some limitations on therapeutic effectiveness: the "burnout syndrome" in psychoanalysts. *Psychoanalytic Quarterly* 55:576–598.

———— (1990). The future of psychoanalysis. *Psychoanalytic Quarterly* 59:177–196.

———— (1995). Discussion: on empirical research. In *Research in Psychoanalysis: Process, Development, Outcome*, ed. T. Shapiro and R. N. Emde. Madison, CT: International Universities Press.

Cremerius, J. (1986). Spurensicherung. Die "Psychoanalytische Bewegung" und das Elend der psychoanalytischen Institution. *Psyche* 12:1063–1091.

———— (1987). Wenn wir als Psychoanalytiker die psychoanalytische Ausbildung organisieren, müssen wir sie psychoanalytisch organisieren! *Psyche* 13:1067–1096.

————, ed. (1995). *The Future of Psychoanalysis*. London: Open Gate, 1999.

Danto, E. A. (1998). The ambulatorium: Freud's free clinic in Vienna. *International Journal of Psycho-Analysis*, 79:287–300.

Debell, D. (1963). A critical digest of the literature on psychoanalytic supervision. *Journal of the American Psychoanalytic Association* 11:546–575.

Deutsch, H. (1932). The training institute and the clinic. *International Journal of Psycho-Analysis*, 13:255–257.

DpG/Deutsche psychoanalytische Gesellschaft (1930). *Zehn Jahre Berliner psychoanalytisches Institut (Poliklinik und Lehranstalt)*. Vienna: Internationaler Psychoanalytisches Verlag.

Dewald, P. A. (1997). A psychoanalytic retrospective. In *More Analysts at Work*, ed. J. Reppen. Northvale, NJ: Jason Aronson.

Dorn, R. M. (1969). Psychoanalysis and psychoanalytic education: What kind of "journey"? *Psychoanalytic Forum* 3:239–254.

———— (1982–83). Training analyst selection: the need for criteria. *International Journal of Psychoanalytic Psychotherapy* 9:691–704.

Dreyfus, H. L., and Dreyfus, S. E. (1986). *Mind over Machine: The Power of Human Intuition and Expertise in the Era of the Computer*. New York: Free Press 1988.

Dulchin, J., and Segal, A. J. (1982a). The ambiguity of confidentiality in a psychoanalytic institute. *Psychiatry* 45:13–25.

———— (1982b). Third party confidences: the uses of information in a psychoanalytic institute. *Psychiatry* 45:27–37.

Dunn, J. (1995). Intersubjectivity in psychoanalysis: a critical review. *International Journal of Psycho-Analysis* 76:723–738.

Eisendorfer, A. (1959). The selection of candidates applying for psychoanalytic training. *Psychoanalytic Quarterly* 28:374–378.

Eisold, K. (1994). The intolerance of diversity in psychoanalytic institutes. *International Journal of Psycho-Analysis* 75:785–800.

———— (1997). Freud as leader: the early years of the Viennese Society. *International Journal of Psycho-Analysis* 78:87–104.

———— (1998). The splitting of the New York Society and the construction of psychoanalytic authority. *International Journal of Psycho-Analysis* 79:871–885.

Eissler, K. (1969). Irreverent remarks about the present and the future of psychoanalysis. *International Journal of Psycho-Analysis* 50:461–471.

Eitingon, M. (1923). Report of the Berlin psycho-analytical polyclinic. *International Journal of Psycho-Analysis* 4:254–268.

———— (1925). Opening address concerning analytical training at the Ninth Psycho-Analytical Congress on September 3, 1925 in Bad Homburg. *International Journal of Psycho-Analysis* 7:129–134.

Ekstein, R., and Wallerstein, R. S. (1958). *The Teaching and Learning of Psychotherapy*, 2nd ed. New York: International Universities Press, 1972.

Elliott, A., and Spezzano, C. (2000a). Psychoanalysis at its limits: navigating the postmodern turn. In *Psychoanalysis at Its Limits: Navigating the Postmodern Turn*, ed. A. Elliott & C. Spezzano. London: Free Association Books.

Elliott, A., and Spezzano, C., eds. (2000b). *Psychoanalysis at Its Limits: Navigating the Postmodern Turn*. London: Free Association Books.

Ellman, S. J. (1996). An analyst at work. In *More Analysts at Work*, ed. J. Reppen. Northvale, NJ: Jason Aronson.

Epstein, R. (1997). Why shrinks have so many problems. *Psychology Today* July/August 1997:59–78.

Etchegoyen, R. H., and Miller, J.-A. (1996). *Silence brisé. Entretien sur le mouvement psychanalytique*. Paris: Agalma/Seuil.

Falzeder, E. (2000). Profession—psychoanalyst: a historical view. *Psychoanal. and History* 2:37–60.

Faure-Pragier, S. (1999). Our training: Does it meet the needs of our candidates? *Psychoanalysis in Europe: Bulletin of the EPF* 52:73–85.

Ferber, L., and Krent, J. (1976). Open forum: the role of the psychoanalyst in a changing society. *International Journal of Psycho-Analysis* 57:441–449.

Ferenczi, S. (1928). The problem of the termination of the analysis. In *Final Contributions to the Problems & Methods of Psycho-Analysis*. New York: Basic Books, 1955.

Ferenczi, S., and Rank, O. (1924). *Entwicklungsziele der Psycho-analyse*. Leipzig: Internationaler Psychoanalytischer Verlag.

Feyerabend, P. (1975). *Against Method: Outline of an Anarchistic Theory of Knowledge*. London: Verso, 1978.

Fischer, N. (1982). Panel Report: Beyond lay analysis: pathways to a psychoanalytic career. *Journal of the American Psychoanalytic Association* 30:701–715.

Fleming, J., and Benedek, T. (1964). Supervision: a method of teaching psychoanalysis. *Psychoanalytic Quarterly* 33:71–96.

Fleming, J., and Weiss, S. S. (1978). Assessment of progress in a training analysis. *International Review of Psycho-Analysis* 5:33–43.

Fliess, R. (1942). Metapsychology of the analyst. *Psychoanalytic Quarterly* 11:211–227.

Fogel, G., and Glick, R. (1991). The analyst's post-graduate development—rereading Freud and working theory through. *Psychoanalytic Quarterly* 60:396–425.

Freedman, N., and Sanville, J. (1999). The confederation of independent psychoanalytic societies in the United States. *International Psychoanalysis. The Newsletter of the IPA* 8/2:46–49.

Freud, A. (1936). The ego and the mechanisms of defense. In *The Writings of Anna Freud*, II. New York: International Universities Press, 1966.

——— (1950 [1938]). The problem of training analysis. In *The Writings of Anna Freud* 4: pp. 407–421. New York: International Universities Press, 1968.

——— (1971). The ideal psychoanalytic institute: a utopia. *Bulletin of the Menninger Clinic* 35:225–239.

——— (1983). Some observations. In *International Psycho-Analytical Association Monograph Series Number 2: The Identity of the Psychoanalyst*, ed. E. Joseph and D. Widlöcher. New York: International Universities Press.

Freud, S. (1900). The interpretation of dreams. *S.E.* 2.

——— (1905). Three essays on the theory of sexuality *S.E.* 7.

——— (1912). Recommendations to physicians practising psychoanalysis. *S.E.* 12.

——— (1914a). On narcissism. *S.E.* 14.

——— (1914b). On the history of the psycho-analytic movement. *S.E.* 14.

——— (1915). The unconscious. *S.E.* 14.

——— (1917). Mourning and melancholia. *S.E.* 14.

——— (1919). Lines of advance in psychoanalytic therapy. *S.E.* 17.

——— (1920). Beyond the pleasure principle. *S.E.* 18.

——— (1921). Group psychology and the analysis of the ego. *S.E.* 18.

——— (1923a). Two encyclopaedia articles. *S.E.* 18.

——— (1923b). The ego and the id. *S.E.* 19.

——— (1926). The question of lay analysis. *S.E.* 20.

——— (1930). Civilization and its discontents. *S.E.* 21.

——— (1933). New introductory lectures on psycho-analysis. *S.E.* 22.

————— (1937). Analysis terminable and interminable. *S.E.* 23.

Frosch, S. (1997). *For and Against Psychoanalysis*. London: Routledge.

————— (1998). Psychoanalysis, science and "truth." In *Freud 2000*, ed. A. Elliott. Cambridge: Polity.

Gedo, J. E. (1979). A psychoanalyst reports at mid-career. *American Journal of Psychiatry* 36:646–649.

————— (1996). The reveries of a solitary scribbler. In *Writing in Psychoanalysis*, ed. E. Piccioli, P. R. Rossi, and A. A. Semi. London: Karnac.

Gerson, B. (1996). *The Therapist as a Person: Life Crises, Life Choices, Life Experiences, and Their Effects on Treatment*. Hillsdale, NJ: Analytic Press.

Giovacchini, P. L. (1985). An analyst at work: reflections. In *Analysts at Work: Practice, Principles, and Technique*, ed. J. Reppen. Northvale, NJ: Jason Aronson, 1994.

Gitelson, M. (1948). Problems of psychoanalytic training. *Psychoanalytic Quarterly* 17:198–211.

————— (1951). Psychoanalysis and dynamic psychiatry. *American Medical Association Archives of Neurology and Psychiatry* 16:280–288.

————— (1954). Therapeutic problems in the analysis of the "normal" candidate. *International Journal of Psycho-Analysis* 35:174–183.

————— (1956). Psychoanalyst, U.S.A., 1955. *American Journal of Psychiatry* 112:700–705.

————— (1962a). The curative factors in psycho-analysis. *International Journal of Psycho-Analysis* 43:194–205.

————— (1962b). The place of psychoanalysis in psychiatric training. *Bulletin of the Menninger Clinic* 26:57–72.

————— (1963). Presidential address, 23rd International Psycho-Analytical Congress: On the present scientific and social position of psycho-analysis. *Bulletin of the International Psychoanalytical Association* 44:521–527.

Glick, R., Eagle, P., Luber, B., and Roose, S. (1996). The fate of training cases. *International Journal of Psycho-Analysis* 77:803–812.

Glover, E. (1927). Lectures on technique in psycho-analysis. *International Journal of Psycho-Analysis* 8:311–338.

————— (1939). Report of the International Training Commission. *International Journal of Psycho-Analysis* 20:212–213.

————— (1968). *The Birth of the Ego*. London: Allen & Unwin.

Goldberg, C. (1992). *The Seasoned Psychotherapist: Triumph over Adversity*. New York: Norton.

Greben, S. E. (1975). Some difficulties and satisfactions inherent in the practice of psychoanalysis. *International Journal of Psycho-Analysis* 56:427–434.

———— (1982–1983). Some sources of conflict within psychoanalytic societies. *International Journal of Psychoanalytic Psychotherapy* 9:657–673.

Greenacre, P. (1961). A critical digest of the literature on selection of candidates for psychoanalytic training. *Psychoanalytic Quarterly* 30:28–55.

———— (1966). Problems of training analysis. *Psychoanalytic Quarterly* 35:540–567.

Greenson, R. R. (1966). That "impossible" profession. *Journal of the American Psychoanalytic Association* 14:9–27.

———— (1967). *The Technique and Practice of Psychoanalysis: Vol. I*. London: Hogarth, 1973.

———— (1969). Origin and fate of new ideas in psychoanalysis. *International Journal of Psycho-Analysis* 50:503–515.

Grinberg, L. (1963). Relations between psycho-analysts. *International Journal of Psycho-Analysis* 44:362–367.

———— (1970). The problems of supervision in psychoanalytic education. *International Journal of Psycho-Analysis* 51:371–383.

———— (1989). Integrity and ethics in "becoming a psychoanalyst." In *The Psychoanalytic Core*, ed. H. P. Blum, E. M. Weinshel, and F. R. Rodman. Madison, CT: International Universities Press.

Grossman, W. I. (1995). Psychological vicissitudes of theory in clinical work. *International Journal of Psycho-Analysis* 76:885–899.

Grotstein, J. (1985). Random notes on the art and science of psychoanalysis from an analyst at work. In *Analysts at Work*, ed. J. Reppen. Northvale, NJ: Jason Aronson, 1994.

Guttman, S. A. (1985). The psychoanalytic point of view: basic concepts and deviant theories. A brief communication. *International Journal of Psycho-Analysis* 66:167–170.

Haesler, L. (1993). Adequate distance in the relationship between supervisor and supervisee. *International Journal of Psycho-Analysis* 74:547–555.

Hagedorn, E. (1992). Die Macht der Lehre und die Ohnmacht der Analyse.

Identifizierung als Konfliktfeld zwischen Analyse und Lehre. In *Lehranalyse und Psychoanalytische Ausbildung*, ed. U. Streeck and H. V. Wethmann. Göttingen: Vandenhoeck & Ruprecht.

Hall, A. (1996). Psychoanalysis, psychoanalytic studies and universities. In *Teaching Transference*, ed. M. Stanton and D. Reason. London: Rebus.

Halmos, P. (1965). *The Faith of the Counsellors*. London: Constable.

Heidegger, M. (1927). *Being and Time*, trans. J. Macquarrie and E. Robinson. New York: Harper & Row, 1962.

Heimann, P. (1954). Problems of the training analysis. *International Journal of Psycho-Analysis* 35:163–168.

——— (1968). The evaluation of applicants for psychoanalytic training—the goals of psychoanalytic education and the criteria for the evaluation of applicants. *International Journal of Psycho-Analysis* 49:527–539.

Herulf, B. (1993). Should we analyze our motives for choosing the profession of analyst? *Bulletin of The European Psychoanalytic Federation* 41:45–51.

Holt, R., and Luborsky, L. (1955). The selection of candidates for psychoanalytic training: on the use of interviews and psychological tests. *Journal of the American Psychoanalytic Association* 3:666–681.

Holzman, P. S. (1976). The future of psychoanalysis and its institutions. *Psychoanalytic Quarterly* 45:250–273.

Interview with Christopher Bollas. (1993). *Psychoanalytic Dialogues* 3:401–430.

Isakower, O. (1939). On the exceptional position of the auditory sphere. *International Journal of Psycho-Analysis* 20:340–348.

Israël, P. (1992). On the adequate distance between supervisor and supervisee: the experience of group supervision in the Paris Psychoanalytic Society. *Bulletin of The European Psychoanalytic Federation* 38:51–59.

——— (1994). Some specific features of the psychoanalytic training. *Bulletin of The European Psychoanalytic Federation* 42:29–37.

Jacobs, T. J. (1985). The use of the self: the analyst and the analytic instrument in the clinical situation. In *Analysts at Work*, ed. J. Reppen. Northvale, NJ: Jason Aronson, 1994.

——— (1999). Countertransference past and present: a review of the concept. *International Journal of Psycho-Analysis* 80:575–594.

Jacoby, R. (1983). *The Repression of Psychoanalysis: Otto Fenichel and the Political Freudians.* Chicago: University of Chicago Press, 1986.

Jones, E. (1937). The future of psycho-analysis. *International Journal of Psycho-Analysis* 17:269–277.

————— (1957). *Sigmund Freud: Life and Work,* Vol. III. London: Hogarth, 1980.

Joseph, E. D. (1978). The ego ideal of the psychoanalyst. *International Journal of Psycho-Analysis* 59:377–386.

————— (1983). Identity of a psychoanalyst. In *Psychotherapy: Impact on Psychoanalytic Training,* ed. E. D. Joseph and R. Wallerstein. New York: International Universities Press.

Joseph, E. D., and Wallerstein. R. eds. (1982). *Psychotherapy: Impact on Psychoanalytic Training. The Influence of the Practice and Theory of Psychotherapy on Education in Psychoanalysis.* New York: International Universities Press.

Kairys, D. (1964). The training analysis: a critical review of the literature and a controversial proposal. *Psychoanalytic Quarterly* 33:485–512.

Kantrowitz, J. (1999). Pathways to self-knowledge: private reflections and mutual supervision and other shared communications. *International Journal of Psycho-Analysis* 80:111–132.

Kappelle, W. (1996). How useful is selection? *International Journal of Psycho-Analysis* 77:1213–1232.

Karon, B. P. (1994). The future of psychoanalysis. In *A History of the Division of Psychoanalysis of the American Psychological Association,* ed. R. C. Lane and M. Meisels. Hillsdale, NJ: Lawrence Erlbaum.

Kelman, H. (1970). The chronic analyst. In *Science and Psychoanalysis,* vol. 16, ed. J. Masserman. New York: Grune & Stratton.

Kernberg, O. (1980). *Internal World and External Reality.* New York: Jason Aronson.

————— (1986). Institutional problems of psychoanalytic education. *Journal of the American Psychoanalytic Association* 34:799–834.

————— (1989). The temptations of conventionality. *International Review of Psycho-Analysis* 16:191–205.

————— (1993). The current status of psychoanalysis. *Journal of the American Psychoanalytic Association* 41:45–62.

————— (1996). Thirty methods to destroy the creativity of psychoanalytic candidates. *International Journal of Psycho-Analysis* 77:1032–1040.

———— (1999). The president's column: present, past, and future: a view from the midpoint. *International Psychoanalysis. The Newsletter of the IPA* 8/1:8–13.

———— (2000). A concerned critique of psychoanalytic education. *International Journal of Psycho-Analysis* 81:97–120.

Kestemberg, E. (1978). In search of a "philosophical" dimension to reflexions on the training of psychoanalysts. *International Journal of Psycho-Analysis* 59:505–509.

King, P. (1983). Identity crises: splits or compromises—adaptive or maladaptive. In *International Psycho-Analytical Association Monograph Series Number 2: The Identity of the Psychoanalyst*, ed. E. Joseph and D. Widlöcher. New York: International Universities Press.

———— (1989). On being a psychoanalyst: integrity and vulnerability in psychoanalytic organizations. In *The Psychoanalytic Core*, ed. H. P. Blum, E. M. Weinshel, and F. R. Rodman. Madison, CT: International Universities Press.

Klauber, J. (1982–1983). Psychoanalytic societies and their discontents. *International Journal of Psychoanalytic Psychotherapy* 9:675–678.

———— (1983). The identity of the psychoanalyst. In *International Psycho-Analytical Association Monograph Series Number 2*, ed. E. Joseph and D. Widlöcher. New York: International Universities Press.

———— (1986). Elements of the psychoanalytic relationship and their therapeutic implications. In *The British School of Psychoanalysis*, ed. G. Kohon. London: Free Association Books.

Knight, R. P. (1953). The present status of organized psychoanalysis in the United States. *Journal of the American Psychoanalytic Association* 1:197–221.

Knowles, M. S. (1973). *The Adult Learner: A Neglected Species*, 3rd ed. Houston: Gulf, 1990.

Kovács, V. (1936). Training and control analysis. *International Journal of Psycho-Analysis* 17:346–358.

Lacan, J. (1978). Proposition du 9 Octobre. *Analytica*, 8.

Lampl-De Groot, J. (1954). Problems of psycho-analytic training. *International Journal of Psycho-Analysis* 35:184–187.

Lane, R. C., and Meisels, M., eds. (1994). *A History of the Division of Psychoanalysis of the American Psychological Association*. Hillsdale, NJ: Lawrence Erlbaum.

Langs, R. (1978). Responses to creativity in psychoanalysts. *International Journal of Psychoanalytic Psychotherapy* 7:189–207.

—— (1997). The framework of supervision in psychoanalytic psychotherapy. In *Supervision and Its Vicissitudes*, ed. B. Martindale et al. London: Karnac.

Laplanche, J., and Pontalis, J.-B. (1967). *The Language of Psycho-Analysis*. London: Hogarth, 1973.

Larsson, B. (1982). The selection and function of the training analyst. *International Review of Psycho-Analysis* 9:381–385.

Laufer, M. E. (1994). Discussion of Paul Israël's paper. *Bulletin of the European Psychoanalytic Federation* 42:38–45.

Lebovici, S. (1978). Presidential address in honour of the centenary of the birth of Karl Abraham. *International Journal of Psycho-Analysis* 59:133–144.

Levenson, E. (1982). Follow the fox. *Contemporary Psychoanalysis* 18:1–15.

Levin, S., and Michaels, J. J. (1961). The participation of psychoanalysts in the medical institutions of Boston. *International Journal of Psycho-Analysis* 42:271–283.

Lewin, B. D., and Ross, H. (1960). *Psychoanalytic Education in the United States*. New York: Norton.

Lifschutz, J. (1976). A critique of reporting and assessment in the training analysis. *Journal of the American Psychoanalytic Association* 24:43–59.

Limentani, A. (1974). The training analyst and the difficulties in the training psychoanalytic situation. *International Journal of Psycho-Analysis* 55:71–77.

—— (1986). Variations on some Freudian themes. *International Journal of Psycho-Analysis* 67:235–243.

—— (1992). What makes training analysis "good enough?" *International Review of Psycho-Analysis* 19:133–135.

Lindgren, U. (1997). Mentorskap och högre utbildning. *Pedagogisk forskning i Sverige* 2:279–289.

Lomas, P. (1987). *The Limits of Interpretation: What's Wrong with Psychoanalysis?* Harmondsworth, UK: Penguin.

—— (1990). On setting up a psychotherapy training scheme. *Free Associations* 20:139–149.

Marmor, J. (1953). The feeling of superiority: an occupational hazard in the practice of psychotherapy. *American Journal of Psychiatry* 110:370–376.

Martin, G. C., Mayerson, P., Olsen, H. E., and Wiberg, J. L. (1978). Candidates' evaluation of psychoanalytic supervision. *Journal of the American Psychoanalytic Association* 26:407–424.

McLaughlin, J. T. (1961). The analyst and the Hippocratic oath. *Journal of the American Psychoanalytic Association* 9:106–123.

―――― (1973). The non-reporting training analyst, the analysis and the institute. *Journal of the American Psychoanalytic Association* 21:697–711.

Meerlo, J. (1952). Some psychological problems in supervision of therapists. *American Journal of Psychotherapy* 6:467–470.

Menninger, K. A. (1942). Presidential address, The American Psychoanalytic Association. *Psychoanalytic Quarterly* 11:287–300.

―――― (1956). Freud and American psychiatry. *Journal of the American Psychoanalytic Association* 4:614–625.

Michels, R. (1988). The future of psychoanalysis. *Psychoanalytic Quarterly* 57:167–185.

Miller, J.-A., ed. (1977). L'excommunication. La communauté psychanalytique en France II. Supplement au numéro 8 d'*Ornicar?*, *Bulletin périodique du Champ freudien*.

Minimal standards for the training of physicians in psychoanalysis. (1956). *Bulletin of the American Psychoanalytic Association* 12:714–721.

Molino, A., ed. (1997). *Freely Associated: Encounters in Psychoanalysis with Christopher Bollas, Joyce McDougall, Michael Eigen, Adam Phillips, Nina Coltart*. London: Free Association Press.

Morrison, N. K., and Evaldson, J. R. (1990). Thoughts on the process of psychoanalytic writing. *Contemporary Psychoanalysis* 26:408–419.

Müller-Braunschweig, C. (1935). Reports of the International Training Commission: Berlin psycho-analytic institute. *International Journal of Psycho-Analysis* 16:246–250.

Nacht, S. (1954). The difficulties of didactic psycho-analysis in relation to therapeutic psycho-analysis. *International Journal of Psycho-Analysis* 35:250–253.

―――― (1962). The curative factors in psycho-analysis. *International Journal of Psycho-Analysis* 43:206–211.

Nielsen, N. (1954). The dynamics of training analysis. *International Journal of Psycho-Analysis* 35:247–249.

Norman, H. F., Blacker, K. H., Oremland, J. D., and Barrett, W. G. (1976). The fate of the transference neurosis after termination of a satisfactory analysis. *Journal of the American Psychoanalytic Association* 24:471–498.

Nosek, L., and Lemlij, M. (1997). Interview with Leo Rangell. *International Psychoanalysis. The Newsletter of the IPA* 6/1.

Oberndorf, C. P. (1926). The Berlin Psychoanalytic Polyclinic. *Psychoanalytic Review* 13:318–322.

Ödman, P.-J. (1995). *Kontrastemas spel. En svensk mentalitets–och pedagogikhistoria*. Stockholm: Prisma, 1998.

Ogden, T. H. (1979). On projective identification. *International Journal of Psycho-Analysis* 60:357–373.

——— (1996). Reconsidering three aspects of psychoanalytic technique. *International Journal of Psycho-Analysis* 77:883–899.

Olinick, S., Warren, S. P., Grigg, K. A., and Granatir, W. I. (1973). The psychoanalytic work ego: process and interpretation. *International Journal of Psycho-Analysis* 54:143–151.

Orgel, S. (1978). Report from the seventh pre-Congress on training. *International Journal of Psycho-Analysis* 59:511–515.

——— (1982). The selection and function of the training analyst in North America. *International Review of Psycho-Analysis* 9:417–434.

——— (1990). The future of psychoanalysis. *Psychoanalytic Quarterly* 59:1–20.

Ornstein, P. H. (1967). Selected problems in learning how to analyze. *International Journal of Psycho-Analysis* 48:448–461.

Parker, I. (1997). *Psychoanalytic Culture: Psychoanalytic Discourse in Western Culture*. London: Sage.

Parsons, M. (1984). Psychoanalysis as vocation and martial art. *International Review of Psycho-Analysis* 11:453–462.

——— (1992). The refinding of theory in clinical practice. *International Journal of Psycho-Analysis* 73:103–115.

Pfeffer, A. (1963). The meaning of the analyst after analysis: a contribution to the theory of therapeutic results. *Journal of the American Psychoanalytic Association* 11:229–244.

——— (1974). The difficulties of the training analyst in the training analysis. *International Journal of Psycho-Analysis* 55:79–83.

Poland, W. S. (1985). At work. In *Analysts at Work*, ed. J. Reppen. Northvale, NJ: Jason Aronson, 1994.

Pollock, G. (1961). Historical perspectives in the selection of candidates for psychoanalytic training. *Psychoanalytic Quarterly* 30:481–496.

————— (1976). Chicago selection research: the selection process and the selector. *Annals of Psychoanalysis* 4:309–331.

Pulver, S. (1985). Psychoanalytic technique: some personal reflections. In *Analysts at Work*, ed. J. Reppen. Northvale, NJ: Jason Aronson, 1994.

Rangell, L. (1967). Psychoanalysis—a current look. *Bulletin of the American Psychoanalytic Association* 23:423–431.

————— (1974). A psychoanalytic perspective leading currently to the syndrome of the compromise of integrity. *International Journal of Psycho-Analysis* 55:3–12.

————— (1982). Transference to theory: the relationship of psychoanalytic education to the analyst's relationship to psychoanalysis. *Annual of Psychoanalysis* 10:29–56.

————— (1988). The future of psychoanalysis: the scientific crossroads. *Psychoanalytic Quarterly* 57:313–340.

Raymond, L. W., and Rosbrow-Reich, S., eds. (1997). *The Inward Eye: Psychoanalysts Reflect on their Lives and Work*. Hillsdale, NJ: Analytic Press.

Reed, G. S. (1994). *Transference Neurosis and Psychoanalytic Experience: Perspectives on Contemporary Clinical Practice*. New Haven, CT: Yale University Press.

Reeder, J. (1996). *Reflecting Psychoanalysis. Narrative and Resolve in the Psychoanalytic Experience*. London: Karnac, 2002.

————— (1998a). Den psykoanalytiska institutionens födelse. *Bulletin of the Swedish Psychoanalytical Association* 50:7–16.

————— (1998b). Dialogiskt tolkande. psykoanalytiska handlingar ur ett hermeneutiskt perspektiv. *Divan* 1–2/1998:53–64.

————— (1998c). Hermeneutics and intersubjectivity: the interpreting dialogue. *Int. Forum Psychoanal.* 7:65–75.

————— (1998d). Kan psykoanalysens kris bli dess räddning? *Bulletin of the Swedish Psychoanalytical Association* 51:44–53.

————— (1999). Från kunskap till kompetens. Reflektioner kring det teoretiska arbetet. *Divan* 3–4/99:10–21.

————— (2002). From knowledge to competence: reflections on theoretical work. *International Journal of Psycho-Analysis* 83:799–809.

Reich, A. (1941). Abstract of "Ober Trophäe Und Triumph" (Trophy and Triumph.) by Otto Fenichel. *Psychoanalytic Quarterly* 10:355–356.

Reiser, M. (1989). The future of psychoanalysis in academic psychiatry: plain talk. *Psychoanalytic Quarterly* 58:185–209.

RHDC. (1995). Report from the House of Delegates Committee on "The Actual Crisis of Psychoanalysis: Challenges and Perspectives." *Internal work paper of the IPA.*

Richards, A. D. (1990). The future of psychoanalysis: the past, present, and future of psychoanalytic theory. *Psychoanalytic Quarterly,* 59:347–369.

———— (1997). Growing up orthodox. In *More Analysts at Work,* ed. J. Reppen. Northvale, NJ: Jason Aronson.

Rickman, J. (1951). Reflections on the function and organization of a psychoanalytical society. *International Journal of Psycho-Analysis* 32:218–237.

Ricoeur, P. (1965). *Freud and Philosophy: An Essay on Interpretation.* New Haven, CT: Yale University Press, 1970.

Riesman, D. (1950). The themes of work and play in the structure of Freud's thought. *Psychiatry* 13:1–16.

Roazen, P. (1969). *Brother Animal: The Story of Freud and Tausk.* New York: Vintage Books, 1971.

———— (1971). *Freud and His Followers.* New York: Da Capo, 1992.

———— (1992). The historiography of psychoanalysis. In *Psychoanalysis in Its Cultural Context: Austrian Studies III,* ed. E. Timms and R. Robertson. Edinburgh: Edinburgh University Press.

Rodrigues, J. (1999). IFPS—is there a difference? *International Forum of Psychoanalysis* 8:268–272.

Rosenbloom, S. (1992). The development of the work ego in the beginning analyst: thoughts on identity formation of the psychoanalyst. *International Journal of Psycho-Analysis* 73:117–126.

Rothstein, A. (1980). Psychoanalytic paradigms and their narcissistic investment. *Journal of the American Psychoanalytic Association* 28:385–395.

Roudinesco, E. (1993). *Jacques Lacan: esquisse d'une vie, histoire d'un système de pensée.* Paris: Fayard.

———— (1997). Psychoanalysis at the end of the 20th century. The situation in France: clinical and institutional prospects. *International Psychoanalysis. The Newsletter of the IPA* 6/1. http://eseries.ipa. org.uk/prev/newsletter/97-1/roudin.htm

Roudinesco, E., and Plon, M. (1997). *Dictionnaire de la psychanalyse.* Paris: Fayard.

Roustang, F. (1976). *Dire Mastery: Discipleship from Freud to Lacan.* Baltimore: Johns Hopkins University Press, 1982.

Rustin, M, (1985). The social organization of secrets: Towards a sociology of psychoanalysis. *International Review of Psycho-Analysis* 12:143–159.

Sachs, D. M. (1992). What makes a training analysis "good enough"?: Freud's science and the synchretistic dilemma. *International Review of Psycho-Analysis* 19:147–157.

Sachs, H. (1947). Observations of a training analyst. *Psychoanalytic Quarterly* 16:147–168.

Sandler, A.-M. (1982). The selection and function of the training analyst in Europe. *International Review of Psycho-Analysis* 9:386–398.

Sandler, J. (1960). On the concept of superego. *Psychoanalytic Study of the Child* 15:128–162. New York: International Universities Press.

———— (1983). Reflections on some relations between psychoanalytic concepts and psychoanalytic practice. *International Journal of Psycho-Analysis* 64:35–45.

———— (1998). Interview with Joseph Sandler. *International Psychoanalysis. The Newsletter of the IPA* 7/1.

Sandler, J., and Dreher, A. U. (1996). *What do Psychoanalysts Want? The Problem of Aims in Psychoanalytic Therapy.* London: Routledge.

Sandler, J., Holder, A., and Meers, D. (1963). The ego ideal and the ideal self. *Psychoanalytic Study of the Child* 18:139–158. New York: International Universities Press.

Schachter, J., and Luborsky, L. (1998). Who's afraid of psychoanalytical research?: Analysts' attitudes towards reading clinical versus empirical research papers. *International Journal of Psycho-Analysis* 79:965–969.

Schafer, R. (1960). The loving and beloved superego in Freud's structural theory. *Psychoanalytic Study of the Child* 15:163–188. New York: International Universities Press.

———— (1979). On becoming a psychoanalyst of one persuasion or another. *Contemporary Psychoanalysis* 15:345–360.

———— (1983). *The Analytic Attitude.* London: Hogarth.

———— (1994). One perspective on the Freud–Klein controversies. *International Journal of Psycho-Analysis* 75:359–365.

———— (1997a). *Tradition and Change in Psychoanalysis.* London: Karnac.

———— (1997b). Current trends in psychoanalysis in the USA, 1997. *International Psychoanalysis. The Newsletter of the IPA* 7/2.

Schneider, A. Z., and Desmond, H. (1994). The psychoanalytic lawsuit: expanding opportunities for psychoanalytic training and practice. In *A History of the Division of Psychoanalysis of the American Psychological Association*, ed. R. C. Lane and M. Meisels. Hillsdale, NJ: Lawrence Erlbaum.

Schön, D. A. (1983). *The Reflective Practitioner: How Professionals Think in Action*. Aldershot, UK: Arena, 1991.

——— (1987). *Educating the Reflective Practitioner*. San Francisco: Jossey-Bass.

Selander, U-B., and Selander, S. (1989). *Professionell handledning*. Lund, Sweden: Studentlitteratur, 1998.

Shapiro, D. (1974). The training setting in training analysis: a retrospective view of the evaluative and reporting role and other "hampering" factors. *International Journal of Psycho-Analysis* 55:297–306.

——— (1976). The analyst's own analysis. *Journal of the American Psychoanalytic Association* 24:5–42.

Shapiro, T., and Emde, R. N., eds. (1995). *Research in Psychoanalysis: Process, Development, Outcome*. Madison, CT: International Universities Press.

Sharpe, E. F. (1947). The psycho-analyst. *International Journal of Psycho-Analysis* 28:1–6.

Shevrin, H. (1981a). The supervision and treatment as seen from the analyst's perspective. In *Becoming a Psychoanalyst*, ed. R. Wallerstein. New York: International Universities Press.

——— (1981b). On being the analyst supervised: return to a troubled beginning. In *Becoming a Psychoanalyst*, ed. R. Wallerstein. New York: International Universities Press.

Silverman, M. (1985). Countertransference and the myth of the perfectly analyzed analyst. *Psychoanalytic Quarterly* 54:175–199.

Skovholt, T. M., and Rønnestad, M. H. (1992). *The Evolving Professional Self: Stages and Themes in Therapist and Counselor Development*. Chichester, UK: Wiley, 1995.

Slap, J. W. (1996). Staying afloat in the paradigmatic flux. In *More Analysts at Work*, ed. J. Reppen. Northvale, NJ: Jason Aronson, 1997.

Slavin, J. (1992). Unintended consequences of psychoanalytic training. *Contemporary Psychoanalysis* 28:616–630.

——— (1994). Professional identity in transition: psychoanalytic education and training in the Division of Psychoanalysis. In *A History of the Division of Psychoanalysis of the American Psychological Association*, ed. R. C. Lane and M. Meisels. Hillsdale, NJ: Lawrence Erlbaum.

———— (1997). Models of learning and psychoanalytic institutions: Can reform be sustained in psychoanalytic training? *Psychoanalytic Dialogues* 7:803–817.

Smirnoff, V. N. (1980). Minimal standards or great expectations? The acceptance of new members to a psychoanalytical society. *EPF Monographs*, 1983.

Spence, D. P. (1997). Case reports and the reality they represent: the many faces of *Nachträglichkeit*. In *The Presentation of Case Material in Clinical Discourse*, ed. I. Ward. London: Freud Museum.

Spruiell, V. (1984). The analyst at work. *International Journal of Psycho-Analysis* 65:13–30.

———— (1989). The future of psychoanalysis. *Psychoanalytic Quarterly* 58:1–28.

Spurling, L. (1997). Using the case study in the assessment of trainees. In *The Presentation of Case Material in Clinical Discourse*, ed. I. Ward. London: Freud Museum.

Stanton, M., and Reason, D. (1996). *Teaching Transference: On the Foundations of Psychoanalytic Studies*. London: Rebus.

Stein, M. H. (1988a). Writing about psychoanalysis: analysts who write and those who do not. *Journal of the American Psychoanalytic Association* 36:105–124.

———— (1988b). Writing about psychoanalysis: analysts who write, patients who read. *Journal of the American Psychoanalytic Association* 36:393–408.

Steiner, R. (1985). Some thoughts about tradition and change arising from an examination of the British Psychoanalytic Society's controversial discussions (1943–1944). *International Review of Psycho-Analysis* 12:27–71.

Steltzer, J. (1986). The formation and deformation of identity during psychoanalytic training. *Free Associations* 7:59–74.

Stensson, J. (1993). Explicit and hidden objectives of the process of training psychoanalysis: panel. *International Forum of Psychoanalysis* 2:52–54.

Stoller, R. (1985). *Observing the Erotic Imagination*. New Haven, CT: Yale University Press.

Stoltenberg, C. D., and Delworth, U. (1987). *Supervising Counselors and Therapists. A Developmental View*. San Francisco: Jossey-Bass.

Stone, L. (1975). Some problems and potentialities of present-day psychoanalysis. *Psychoanalytic Quarterly* 44:331–369.

Stout, C. E. (1993). *From the Other Side of the Couch: Candid Conversations with Psychiatrists and Psychologists*. Westport, CT: Greenwood.

Strachey, J. (1934). The nature of the therapeutic interaction of psychoanalysis. *International Journal of Psycho-Analysis* 15:127–159.

Sutherland, J. D. (1980). The British object relations theorists: Balint, Winnicott, Fairbairn, Guntrip. *Journal of the American Psychoanalytic Association* 28:829–860.

Symington, N. (1986). *The Analytic Experience*. London: Free Association Books.

Szalita, A. (1968). Reanalysis. *Contemporary Psychoanalysis* 4:83–102.

Szasz, T. S. (1958). Psycho-analytic training—a socio-psychological analysis of its history and present status. *International Journal of Psycho-Analysis* 39:598–611.

Szecsödy, I. (1994). Supervision—a complex tool for psychoanalytic training. *Scandinavian Psychoanalytic Review* 17:119–129.

—— (1996). *Report from the Committee on "Evaluation of Different Training Models"* of the House of Delegates. Mimeographed.

—— (1997). (How) Is learning possible in supervision? In *Supervision and Its Vicissitudes*, ed. B. Martindale et al. London: Karnac.

Terman, D. M. (1972). Summary of the candidates' pre-congress conference, Vienna, 1971. *International Journal of Psycho-Analysis* 53:47–48.

Thickstun, J. T. (1985). An analyst at play. In *Analysts at Work*, ed. J. Reppen. Northvale, NJ: Jason Aronson, 1994.

Thomä, H. (1993). Training analysis and psychoanalytic education: proposals for reform. *The Annual of Psychoanalysis* 21:3–75.

Thomä, H., and Kächele, H. (1999). Memorandum on a reform of psychoanalytic education. *International Psychoanalysis. The Newsletter of the IPA* 8/2:33–35.

Thompson, C. (1958). A study of the emotional climate of psychoanalytic institutes. *Psychiatry* 21:45–51.

Torras de Beà, E. (1992). Towards a "good-enough" training analysis. *International Review of Psycho-Analysis* 19:159–167.

Treurniet, N. (1993). What is psychoanalysis now? *International Journal of Psycho-Analysis* 74:873–891.

van der Leeuw, P. J. (1962). Symposium: selection criteria for the training of psycho-analytic students. *International Journal of Psycho-Analysis* 43:277–281.

———— (1968). The psychoanalytic society. *International Journal of Psycho-Analysis* 49:160–164.

Wagner, P. S. (1963). The second analysis. *International Journal of Psycho-Analysis* 44:481–489.

Wallerstein, R. S. (1972). The futures of psychoanalytic education. *Journal of the American Psychoanalytic Association* 20:591–606.

———— (1978). Perspectives on psychoanalytic training around the world. *International Journal of Psycho-Analysis* 59:477–504.

———— (1981a). The psychoanalyst's life: expectations, vicissitudes, and reflections. *International Review of Psycho-Analysis* 8:285–298.

————, ed. (1981b). *Becoming a Psychoanalyst: A Study of Psychoanalytic Supervision*. New York: International Universities Press.

———— (1988). One psychoanalysis or many? *International Journal of Psycho-Analysis* 69:5–21.

———— (1992). Final summary statement, International Scientific Colloquium on the Therapeutic Process in Child and Adult Analysis. *Bulletin of the Anna Freud Centre* 15:173–82.

———— (1997). Förord. In *Supervision and Its Vicissitudes*, ed. B. Martindale et al. London: Karnac.

———— (1998a). The IPA and the American Psychoanalytic Association: a perspective on the regional association agreement. *International Journal of Psycho-Analysis* 79:553–564.

———— (1998b). *Lay Analysis: Life Inside the Controversy*. Hillsdale, NJ: Analytic Press.

Wallerstein, R. S., and Fonagy, P. (1999). Psychoanalytic research and the IPA: history, present status and future potential. *International Journal of Psycho-Analysis* 80:91–109.

Wallerstein, R. S., and Weinshel, E. M. (1989). The future of psychoanalysis. *Psychoanalytic Quarterly* 58:341–373.

Weigert, E. (1955). Special problems in connection with termination of training analyses. *Journal of the American Psychoanalytic Association* 3:630–640.

Weinshel, E. M. (1982). The functions of the training analysis and the selection of the training analyst. *International Review of Psycho-Analysis* 9:434–444.

Weiss, S. S. (1982). The problem of the problem candidate: a significant issue for psychoanalytic educators. *Annual of Psychoanalysis* 10:77–92.

Weiss, S. S., and Fleming, J. (1975). Evaluation of progress in supervision. *Psychoanalytical Quarterly* 44:191–205.

Wellendorf, F. (1995). Learning from experience and the experience of learning: reflections on the psychoanalytical training. *International Forum of Psychoanalysis* 4:137–148.

Wheelis, A. (1956). The vocational hazards of psycho-analysis. *International Journal of Psycho-Analysis* 37:171–184.

Widlöcher, D. (1978). The ego ideal of the psychoanalyst. *International Journal of Psycho-Analysis* 59:387–390.

——— (1983). Psychoanalysis today: a problem of identity. In *International Psycho-Analytical Monograph Series Number 2: The Identity of the Psychoanalyst*, ed. E. Joseph and D. Widlöcher. New York: International Universities Press.

Winnicott, D. W. (1958). The capacity to be alone. In *The Maturational Processes and the Facilitating Environment*. New York: International Universities Press, 1965.

Winter, S. (1999). *Freud and the Institution of Psychoanalytic Knowledge*. Stanford, CA: Stanford University Press.

Zemke, R., and Zemke, S. (1995). Adult learning: What do we know for sure? *Training* June:31–40.

Zinberg, N. E. (1967). Psycho-analytic training and psycho-analytic values. *International Journal of Psycho-Analysis* 48:88–96.

Index

Aarons, Z. A., 90, 158, 164, 186, 205
Abraham, K., 62
Adler, A., 69
Alexander, F., 57
American Psychiatric Association, 73
American Psychoanalytical
    Association (APA), 65, 73–74,
    77–79, 136, 187, 192, 239
American Psychological Association,
    78
Analyzability, 76, 102
Apprenticeship, 135
Aristotle, 16, 42
Arlow, J. A., 87, 106, 113, 118, 138,
    142, 143, 144, 157, 158, 166,
    176, 182, 184, 191, 208, 236
Aryan, 64
Assimilation, 37, 40, 42–45, 50–52,
    89, 107, 108, 115, 209
Average expectable psychoanalyst,
    112

Babcock, C., 115
Bak, R. C., 90, 115, 135, 200, 204
Baker, R., 187
Balint, M., 66–69, 95–100, 103, 105,
    113, 166, 223
Baudry, F. D., 121, 124, 129, 136
Being, 18, 22, 45, 177

Beland, H., 114, 183
Benedek, T., 121, 129, 155, 161
Bergmann, M. S., 197, 204
Berlin
    institute, 8, 56–64, 68, 96, 101,
        119, 125, 229
    polyclinic, 57–59
Berman, E., 124, 235
Bernardi R., 152, 160, 191
Bernfeld, S., 55, 57, 63, 72, 115,
    125, 223, 229
Bibring, E., 119, 124, 126, 136
Bibring, G., 99, 106, 164
Bion, W. R., 34, 43, 116, 215–216
Bird, B., 74, 75, 90, 143
Blitzsten, N. L., 126
Blum, H. P., 199
Boehm, F., 57
Bonaparte, M., 70
Bourdieu, P., 199–200
Brenner, C., 142, 211
British school, 76
Britton, R., 131, 194
Bruzzone, M., 181
Buechler, S., 202

Calef, V., 8, 102, 139, 143, 185, 198,
    204
Candidate. See training candidate.

301

Career
    of the analyst, 157, 197–220, 229
    analyst's inner, 213–214
Character analysis, 96–97, 99, 100
Coalition of Independent
    Psychoanalytic Societies
    (IPS), 78
Coltart, N., 84, 152, 159, 185, 203
Commonsense psychology, 35, 37,
    38, 40, 44, 46, 50–51
Communication, 18, 20, 29, 31
Competence, 36, 51, 202, 245
Complex. See superego
Confidentiality, 102, 111, 150, 180
    breach of, 131, 134–135, 179
Conscience of the analysis, 139. See
    also setting
Construction, 37, 38–42, 50, 188
Control case, 59, 61, 62–63, 119. See
    also supervision
Convoying, 164
Cotransference, 21
Countertransference, 19–21, 115,
    127, 162, 163
Cremerius, J., 56, 94, 142, 156, 157,
    165, 178, 182, 194, 235
Crisis of psychoanalysis, 224, 242–
    247
Curriculum, 61, 62, 64, 67, 71, 166,
    236

Death drive/instinct, 171, 264
DeBell, D., 126
Deconstruction, 37, 39–41, 44, 52
Desmond, H., 78
Destiny, 20, 26, 28, 29
Deutsch, H., 64
Dewald, P. A., 220
Didactic analysis, 59–60, 61, 62, 86,
    94–118. See also training
    analysis
Disposition, 15, 139, 251

Dorn, R. M., 75, 77, 88, 118, 141, 151,
    160, 162, 173, 176, 196, 220
Dulchin, J., 132–134, 157, 179–180,
    181, 186

École freudienne, 70–71
Education, 83
Ego ideal, 167, 168–170, 173, 205,
    213–220
    as narratheme, 215–216
Ego psychology, 70, 72, 76, 77, 93,
    191
Eisendorfer, A., 91, 211
Eitingon, M., 57, 58, 62, 63
Ekstein, R., 124
Elliott, A., 197
Ellman, S. J., 191
Empathy, 140
Empirical foundation, 49, 61, 188
Epoch(s) of the psychoanalytical
    institution, 66–72
    first, 67–68, 85
    second, 68, 85–86, 126
    third, 68–72, 85, 93, 114, 176,
        196, 223–224, 241, 247
Ethic(s), ethical, 52, 55, 112, 139, 237
    dimension of analyst's career, 213
    dimension of self-reflection, 216–
        217
    of care, 28, 110
    of psychoanalysis, 36, 111, 131,
        268
    professional, 104, 111, 216, 268
    sensibility, 174
Ethical failure, 33–34
Ethos, 4, 110, 139, 197, 198, 200,
    201
Evaldson, J. R., 193
Evaluation
    of candidates, 101–106, 119, 123,
        129, 235
    of training analysts, 180

Evenly suspended attention, 27–29, 137

Experience, 37, 45, 48–50, 61, 109, 191
    psychoanalytic, 17–18, 25, 26, 39, 41, 47, 49, 50, 107, 111, 188, 212
    transmission of, 106–112, 137–138

Faith in the Other, 32–33, 110, 250
Falzeder, E., 59
Fantasy, 43
Faure-Pragier, S., 84
Fenichel, O., 57, 63, 206
Ferenczi, S., 97, 98, 106
Figueira, S. A., 191
Fleming, J., 103, 121, 126, 129
Fliess, R., 87–88, 105, 108, 198
Fogel, G., 188, 205
Free associating, 35
Freud, A., 70, 84, 85–86, 94, 117, 142, 163, 176, 177
Freud, S., 18, 28, 41, 46, 47, 56–57, 59, 65, 67, 69, 72, 76, 97–98, 113, 141, 142, 158, 168–172, 176, 189, 190, 191, 199, 210, 214
Frosch, S., 113, 158
Future
    of psychoanalysis, 241–247
    of psychoanalytic institutions, 244–247

Gedo, J. E., 195, 203
Giovacchini, P. L., 206
Gitelson, M., 77, 99, 100, 128, 150
Glick, R., 188, 201, 205
Glover, E., 42–43, 98
Good, the, 15–17, 147, 215, 217, 223, 230
    the good life, 16–17

Greben, S. E., 117, 159, 163, 184, 185, 187
Greenacre, P., 86, 92, 99, 113, 115, 117, 118, 162, 164, 165, 204
Greenson, R. R., 87, 162, 195, 205, 212
Grinberg, L., 8, 124, 136
Grossman, W. I., 45, 190
Grotstein, J., 185, 192
Guttman, S. A., 230
Göring, M. H., 63

Haesler, L., 124, 139
Habitus, 108
Hárnik, J., 57, 63
Hall, A., 141
Hate, 20, 154, 170–172, 223, 264
    culture of, 173–176
    externalized, 176–188
    interpretation as expression of, 208–210
    transmission of, 173, 177, 186
Hegel, 44
Heimann, P., 87, 93, 99, 165
Hermeneutics, hermenutic, 39, 49, 51, 208
    of suspicion, 210–213
Heuristics, 174, 184
Hippocratic oath, 198
Hitler, A., 63
Horney, K., 57, 60, 85
Hypochondria, 44

Identification, 36, 40, 106–108, 115, 116, 138–139, 161, 176
    with the aggressor, 176–177, 183, 206, 211
Identity, 183
    professional, 9, 55, 129, 162
    psychoanalytic, 152, 166, 202
Ideology, 38–40, 46, 71, 76, 121, 183

Immanent pedagogy, 166–168, 173, 174, 186, 198, 201, 207
Indoctrination, 116
Infantilization of the candidate, 115, 163, 234
Institute(s), 84, 124
Institution(s), 56, 67, 100, 154–165
 analyst's relation to, 147–153
 democracy within psycho-
  analytical, 157, 240–241
 future of psychoanalytic, 244–247
 institutional problems, 223–224, 227
 power within, 240–241
 resistance of, 205
Internalization, 107, 173, 177, 201
 of analyst's/supervisor's
  function, 106–109, 139–140
International Psychoanalytic
 Association (IPA), 7, 8, 59, 62,
 64–66, 70–71, 77–79, 96, 114,
 120, 157, 158, 192, 224, 239,
 246
International Federation of
 Psychoanalytic Societies
 (IFPS), 7, 64, 77–78, 246
International Training Committee
 (ITC), 62, 64–66, 68, 97
Interpretation
 as a double-edged sword, 210
 as expression of hate, 208–210
 tyranny of, 208–210
Interpreting, 18, 29–32, 34–35, 43,
 51, 208, 215, 218, 250
Intersubjectivity, 17–18, 19, 29,
 109, 124, 139, 249–250
Intimacy, 128–130, 160
Introjection, 113, 172, 174, 176, 210
Introspection, 43
Inventing the analysand, 50–52

Jewish, 63–66
Jones, E., 63, 66, 72, 117
Joseph, E. D., 8, 218
Jung, C. G., 69

Kairys, D., 103–105, 118, 162, 165
Kappelle, W., 85, 93
Karon, B. P., 79
Kernberg, O., 114, 142, 147, 156,
 158, 181, 182, 187, 191, 193,
 195, 196, 223, 224–226, 235–
 236
King, P., 156, 160, 162, 175, 195,
 203, 205
Klauber, J., 186, 189, 201–202, 204
Klein, M., 70, 76, 115
Kleinian, 108
Knight, R. P., 77, 89, 188
Knowledge, 36, 38, 42, 238, 251
 arrogance of, 190
Knowing, 251
Knowles, M. S., 167
Kovács, V., 97, 125–126, 231

Lacan, J., 70–71, 108–109, 196, 253,
 272
Lagache, D., 70
Lampl, H., 57
Lampl-de Groot, J., 87, 155
Langs, R., 135, 195, 212
Laplanche, J., 106
Lay analyst, lay analysis, 65
Lebovici, S., 173
Lewin, B. D., 102–103
Lifschutz, J., 104
Limentani, A., 115, 117, 204
Lindgren, U., 123
Listening, 29, 107, 210
Love, 20, 28, 38, 147, 154, 170, 172,
 173, 208, 217, 223
Luborsky, L., 142

Marmor, J., 187, 212
Marx, K., 210
Matrix
  of communication, 18–19, 20, 29,
    34, 36, 250
  of transference, 21–23, 29, 31,
    109–110, 120, 127, 137–138,
    140, 250
McLaughlin, F., 217
McLaughlin, J. T., 105, 106
Medicine, 65, 73, 75, 77–79, 200–
  201, 239
Medical paradigm, 72
Meerlo, J., 130
Menninger, K. A., 74
Mental health of psychoanalyst, 152
Mentor, mentorship, 113, 122–123,
  124, 135–140, 219–220
Merit
  recognition of, 157, 230, 239
Metaphysics, metaphysical, 41, 72,
  189
Metapsychology, 37, 39, 45–48, 188
Middle group, 70
Morrison, N. K., 193
Müller-Braunschweig, C., 57, 63
Myth, 42, 47–48, 50, 52

Nacht, S., 99, 117, 162, 203
Narratheme, 214–217
Narrative, 35, 41–42, 47–48, 51,
  214–219
Nielsen, N., 101, 160
Nieto, M., 152, 160, 191
Nietzsche, F., 210
Normality, 90–91, 100, 184
Normalization of the candidate/
  analyst, 112–118, 121, 210

Oberndorf, C. P., 57
Observation, 48–49

Ödman, P.-J., 167
Olinick, S., 15
Orgel, S., 149, 159, 163
Ornstein, P. H., 123, 130, 137
Orthodox, orthodoxy, 112, 149,
  177, 206–208, 211, 241
Other, the, 18, 22, 32–33, 36, 51,
  110, 171, 176, 209, 250

Paranoia, 92, 148, 178–188, 193, 225
Parsons, M., 92
Pedagogic conflict, 121–125
Personal analysis, 92, 94–118, 227,
  228–229
  therapeutic aim of, 95–101
  wholly independent, 230–233
  See also training analysis
Pfeffer, A., 128, 166
Philosophy, 47
  of psychoanalytical education,
    143
Plon, M., 64
Poland, W. S., 213
Pollock, G., 181
Pontalis, J–B., 106
Power, 240–241
  will to, 210
Praxis, 16, 147, 204, 215, 227
Process, the analytical, 109–110
Profession, professional, 61–62, 83,
  89, 90, 104, 143, 197–198, 204,
  227
  development, 125, 129, 198, 201–
    220, 245
  ego, 88
  medical, 56, 199, 201, 239
  superego. See superego
  supervision, 135–136
Professionalism, 88, 143–144, 154
Professionalization, 55–56, 68, 73,
  199, 227

Psychic reality, 22, 40, 41, 46, 47, 50
Psychiatry, 254–255
  dynamic, 74, 76–77, 255
  psychoanalysis and, 72–77, 149, 242, 243
Psychoanalysis
  crisis of, 224, 242–247
  cultural significance of, 73
  future of, 241–247
  nature of the work, 149–150
Psychoanalytic movement, 69, 72, 241, 247
Psychoanalytical attitude, 110, 150–152
Psychoanalytical institution(s), 6, 10, 77, 100, 147
Psychologist(s), 78–79, 239
Psychopath, 90–91, 133
  pursuit of, 178–188
Psychopathology, 90–91, 181, 211
Pulver, S., 8

Radó, S., 57, 59
Rangell, L., 175, 192
Rank, O., 106
Reed, G. S., 191–192, 214
Reflection, 30
  self-, 116, 214–219
Reik, T., 63, 65
Report
  nonreporting system, 126, 132–134, 135
  reporting system, 101–105, 129, 132, 162, 224, 233, 258–259
  supervisor's, 121–122, 135
  to the supervisor, 124–125
Representation, 17, 215, 250
Research, 68, 78, 142, 150, 235–239, 266
  analysis, 98, 100, 187, 188
Respectability, 55, 56, 72, 154

Richards, A. D., 114
Rickman, J., 152, 196
Ricoeur, P., 210
Roazen, P., 190
Ross, H., 102–103
Ross, H., 102
Roudinesco, E., 64
Rustin, M., 134, 149

Sachs, H., 57, 99, 125
Sandler, A.-M., 156, 235
Sandler, J., 187
Schacht, L., 147
Schachter, J., 142
Schafer, R., 194, 207
Schneider, A. Z., 78
Second analysis, 117–118
Segal, A. J., 132–134, 157, 179–180, 181, 186
Selection of candidates, 85–94, 101, 121, 211
Self-analysis, 218
Self-evaluation of the candidate, 105
Setting, 21, 130, 139
  keeper of the analytical, 110–112, 139, 198, 219
Shapiro, D., 100, 102, 161, 164
Silverman, M., 151
Simmel, E., 57, 62, 63
Slavin, J., 183, 207
Smirnoff, V. N., 89
Speculation, 39, 46, 49–50
Spezzano, C., 197
Spruiell, V., 209, 217
Spurling, L., 131, 194
Steiner, R., 39
Steltzer, J., 121, 207–208
Stensson, J., 173
Stoller, R., 184
Stone, L., 93, 189, 195, 196
Strachey, J., 87, 140
Sublation, 44

Superego, 5, 113, 130, 152, 167,
    168–170, 172, 173, 178, 199,
    201, 202, 208, 213–220, 249,
    264
and work ego, 198
as cherished possession, 206
as reservoir of introjected hate,
    172–176, 193
(institutional) superego system, 5,
    117, 153, 174, 177
professional/psychoanalytical
    superego, 4, 6, 153, 173,
    184, 199, 201, 206, 207, 210,
    214, 271
superego complex, 5, 6, 7, 9–11,
    84, 91, 153–154, 165–188,
    196, 204, 205, 223–224, 227,
    241, 244, 247
terror, 212
tyranny of, 172
Supertherapy, 97–99, 232
Supervised case(s)
number and frequency of, 119–
    120
Supervision, 44, 59, 105, 118–140,
    219
as instrument of evaluation, 129,
    132
conflict with training analysis,
    126–128
goals of, 136–137
intimacy and control in, 128–135
frequency of, 136
negative effects of, 122, 135
patient-oriented vs. therapist-
    oriented, 123–125
suggested changes in, 233–235
synchretism of, 125–128
Supervisor, 63, 105, 113, 119, 132,
    233–235
analyst as, 125–126
as mentor, 135–140

candidate's choice of, 120, 234
presence of, 103
training for becoming, 156, 233
Surviving the first years as analyst,
    201–220
Sutherland, J. D., 191
Symington, N., 35
Symptom, 43, 100, 194
Symptom analysis, 96
Syncretism, 102–105, 122
of supervison, 125–128, 234
Szasz, T. S., 64, 67–68, 74, 143
Szecsödy, I., 122, 129, 138, 231

Technique, 51, 59, 112, 121
Technical seminar, 62–63, 141
Theoretical
divergence, 194
seminar, studies 62, 67, 140–144,
    236
work, 35–52, 87, 144, 150, 188–
    197, 219, 235–239
Theory, 36, 43, 115, 141, 144, 187,
    192, 209
clinical, 37, 38–42, 46, 188, 235
Thickstun, J. T., 130
Thomä, H., 114, 115, 118, 126–128,
    148, 158, 165, 182, 235
Thompson, C., 162, 163, 232
Torras de Beà, E., 91, 112
Training, 11, 55, 58, 64, 67–69, 74,
    83–85, 143, 148, 205
accessibility of, 239–240
bipartite model of, 227, 230, 232,
    233
candidate, 60, 84, 178
committee, 62
system of Berlin, 59–64, 229, 236
tripartite model of, 83, 119, 230,
    232
Training analysis, 66–67, 94–118,
    119, 126–128, 132, 165, 166

Training analyst (institution), 60,
    66, 71, 86, 106, 108, 113, 114,
    119, 125, 133, 154–165, 166,
    180
  abolition of, 228–230, 233
  age of, 156
  appointment of, 157–159, 220
  as a class system, 157–160, 180
  candidate's identification with,
    161–164
  dilemma of, 159–160
  family-like relations within, 160–
    165
  requirements of excellence for
    becoming, 154–155
Training institute
  as art academy, 225
  as technical or trade school,
    225
  as monastery or religious retreat,
    225
  as university college, 226, 236
Transference, 19–21, 22, 26, 28, 41,
    107, 140, 211–212
  negative, 25, 97, 165
Truth, 18, 29, 34–35, 43, 49
  and faithfulness, 35, 50

Unconscious, the, 18, 21, 36, 39, 41,
    46, 59, 75, 94, 95, 114, 211
Unconscious content(s), 17, 114
Unsuitability of the candidate, 88–
    91, 101

van der Leeuw, P. J., 8, 85, 88, 166,
    182, 184, 185
Virtue(s), 87, 249
  catalogue(s) of, 87, 88

Wallerstein, R. S., 84, 89,114, 115,
    121, 124, 144, 148, 208, 212
Webster, T., 75
Weigert, E., 98, 162, 166
Weinshel, E., 102, 139, 156, 157,
    163, 176, 185, 198, 204
Weiss, S. S., 103, 121, 178
Weltanschauung, 183, 191, 211
Wheelis, A., 203, 204, 205
Widlöcher, D., 152
Winnicott, D. W., 191
Wish to become an analyst,
    100–101
Work-ego, 87–88, 108, 198–199

Zinberg, N. E., 166

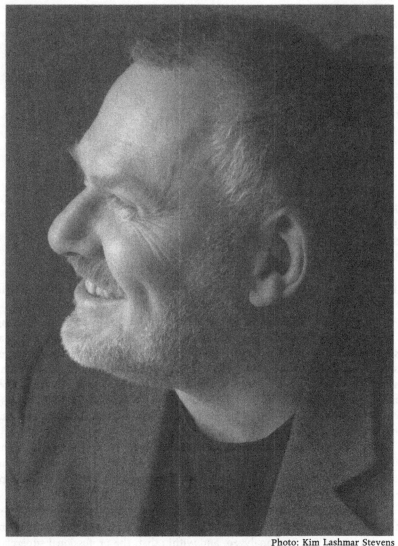

Photo: Kim Lashmar Stevens

JURGEN REEDER was born in 1947. He is a Ph.D., analyst, training analyst, and member of the Swedish Psychoanalytical Association. In private practice since 1979, he is an Associate Professor at the University of Stockholm, Sweden, and the author of *Reflecting Psychoanalysis: Narrative and Resolve in the Psychoanalytic Experience.*

ABSTRACT

Reeder, Jurgen
jurgen.reeder@telia.com

Hate and Love in Psychoanalytic Institutions:
The Dilemma of a Profession

Original title:
Hat och kärlek i psykoanalytiska institutioner
En professions dilemma
Stockholm/Stehag: Brutus Östlings Bokförlag Symposion 2001
Monograph, 397 pages.

Two heuristic concepts are central to this study (comprising also its main hypotheses):

1) *The professional superego*, designating a prescriptive and prohibiting instance incorporated by the individual admitted to a certain occupational sphere. The prescriptive aspect works like a professional ideal and in this respect the superego can be said to sustain a professional "ethos" or spirit. The superego's prohibiting aspect will, however, install an inner observing eye, not only offering necessary protection against detrimental aberrations, but also evoking fantasies of critical or condemning colleagues, thus hampering possibilities of good professional work.

2) *The superego complex* is the wider concept, encompassing both the internalized superego of the individual professional and the structures within institutions that express and promulgate this superego. In addition, the concept seeks to cover their mutual workings.

This study investigates—mainly through a study of the available literature— the superego complex within psychoanalytical institutions. Its structures are charted, described, and analyzed, and within that, the professional superego. In addition are studied the ways of functioning and the forms through which these structures are transmitted and maintained within psychoanalytic training programs and the general analytic societal setting.

The writing of this book was made possible by a research grant from The Swedish Council for Research in the Humanities and Social Sciences.

Printed in the United States
By Bookmasters